SEVERE ME: MORE NOTES FOR CARERS

GREG CROWHURST

Stonebird

Copyright © 2020 by Greg Crowhurst

All rights reserved.

No part of this book may be reproduced in any form or by any electronic or mechanical means, including information storage and retrieval systems, without written permission from the author, except for the use of brief quotations in a book review.

978-1-716-38453-0

Imprint: Lulu.com

HOW MANY?

How many days, weeks, months, years, has the sun, shining outside my window called to me to come out and play,

Yet I have been unable to comply?

How many times has the world passed me by, the simplest of things being impossible to achieve?

How many years have I lain in bed unable to move, speak or get even the simplest most basic need met?

How long have I sat in impossibly twisted painful postures paralysed stiffly, feet glued to the floor too heavy to move?

How many, many thoughts have been lost, barred access to, how many words misspoken or phrases cut short or twisted into unrecognisable form,

Too many to count, too many to tell, too many to remember?

How much pain can one body take, burning, throbbing, itching, screaming, continuously, with no let up, no respite, no remission, no effective treatment?

How much harm has been done to me by ordinary things like insignificant noises, sudden movements, a waft of strong perfume or wrong interventions and unaware people, leaving me lost and broken yet again, with no way out except to strive for inner peace, patience and to wait, of necessity, for it to pass?

How much waiting has been endured, waiting for healing, waiting for an easing of symptoms, waiting for recognition, waiting for the right help, waiting for the right knowledge, waiting for the right way forward, that never comes?

DISCLAIMER

Please note that the publisher and the author cannot be held accountable for any damages or actions arising from reading this book, which is presented for informational purposes only. This book is not intended to be a substitute for the medical advice of a licensed physician. The reader should consult with their doctor in any matters relating to his/her health. Any use of this information is at your own risk. The views of contributors are not necessarily those of the publisher or author, under no circumstances can they be held accountable for any loss or claim arising out of the opinions expressed or suggestions made.

© 2020 Stonebird All rights reserved

This book is dedicated to the memory of our dear friend Merryn Croft [1] who died from ME just after her 21st Birthday and all the other much missed friends who we have known down the years, who have also died with ME. Each kindness is remembered.

Merryn was an incredibly special person, full of love and life. She was enthusiastic, kind and compassionate, incredibly generous and supportive to others, reaching out to them, despite horrendously severe and complex symptoms, that left her bed bound, in terrible untreatable pain, severely noise, light and touch sensitive, enduring intestinal failure, myoclonic seizures and paralysis.

We will never forget her. She was greatly loved by the ME community and will always be remembered. We hold her and her family especially close in our hearts.

We also dedicate this book, with all our love, to Kara Jane Spencer, a very special friend who has touched the whole world with her music and love. [2]

---

1. For more information on Merryn please see: https://stonebird.co.uk/merryn/index.htm
2. Kara's song "Remember Us" is a exceptionally powerful tribute to the struggles of the ME Community and all of those who have died. https://www.youtube.com/watch?v=gfyvQuDt5ZE&feature=emb_logo

ACKNOWLEDGMENTS

∼

Thank you so much to **Jane Collingridge** for permission to publish **Emily's** Appeal and her poem on Pain. A huge thank you to all those who have so kindly contributed to this book:

- **Moira Dillon,** from ME Advocates Ireland (MEAI).
- **Colleen Steckel**, from the USA.
- **Alem Matthees**, and his mother **Helen Donovan**, from Australia.
- **Soph Clark**, from the UK.
- **Christine Fenton**, from ME Advocates Ireland (MEAI).
- **Corina Duyn,** from ME Advocates Ireland (MEAI).
- **Joan McParland,** Treasurer and Founder Hope 4 ME & Fibro Charity, Northern Ireland.
- **Wendy Boutilier**, founder of Global Advocates for Myalgic Encephalomyelitis (GAME), Canada.

- **Eira Stuart,** from the UK.

Above all I cannot thank my wife Linda enough. Compiling this book has been exceptionally difficult. I could not have done it without her support, guidance and contributions to this book, especially her poetry.

CONTENTS

How Many?	1
Disclaimer	3
Acknowledgments	7
1. Overview	13
2. Introduction Moira Dillon from ME Advocates Ireland (MEAI)	15
3. Valuable Resources by Colleen Steckel, ME Patient and Advocate	18
4. Foreword by Greg Crowhurst	20
5. Part One: The Severe/Very Severe ME Experience	23
6. Broken Places	24
7. The Disease Myalgic Encephalomyelitis	26
8. People	32
9. Barriers To Connection	33
10. Neglect in Severe and Very Severe ME	49
11. The Paradox of Caring for People Diagnosed with Severe or Very Severe ME	57
12. My Invisible World	68
13. An Introduction to Severe ME: A Conundrum of Care	84
14. Severe ME A Conundrum In Care by Eira Stuart	85
15. Introduction to The Monstrous Sting In The Tail	94
16. The Monstrous Sting in the Tail of Myalgic Encephalomyelitis by Joan McParland	96
17. Introduction To Accessibility and Creativity: A Review of Into the Light, Artist Book in a Box by Corina Duyn	101
18. Accessibility and Creativity a Review of Into The Light, Artists Book in a Box by Corina Duyn	102
19. Introduction to Emily's appeal.	107

20. An Appeal, by Emily Collingridge	108
21. It Would Not Be So	112
22. When I Can, when I Can't, when I Might, by Linda Crowhurst	115
23. Part Two: Key Symptoms of Severe and Very Severe ME	119
24. How Do You Convey How Very Ill You Are?	120
25. A Symptom Severity Scale	124
26. Experience and Underlying Symptoms	129
27. Dealing With Symptoms	133
28. Issues of Noise, Light, Touch, Chemical and Movement Sensitivity in Severe and Very Severe ME	151
29. Bitter Lands	174
30. The Problem of Paralysis in ME	176
31. What does Paralysis feel like?	182
32. Helpless to Get Help	187
33. Introduction to the Sheer Helplessness of Paralysis, by Christine Fenton	189
34. The Sheer Absolute helplessness of Paralysis, by Christine Fenton	190
35. Contemplate Paralysis If You Can	193
36. Brain Fog in Severe and Very Severe Me	199
37. How To Support Someone With Sleep Dysfunction	202
38. Pain In Very Severe ME	205
39. Introduction to "Pain" poem by Emily Collingridge	208
40. Pain, by Emily Collingridge	209
41. Introduction to My Coping Mechanism by Corina Duyn	212
42. My Coping Mechanism by Corina Duyn	214
43. Useful Symptom Experience Record Chart	216
44. Introduction to Can a Care Plan help to ensure I have a 'Positive Experience of Care'? By Christine Fenton	218
45. Can a Care Plan help to ensure I have a 'Positive Experience of Care'? by Christine Fenton	219

46. Part Three: On the Caring Role	229
47. Vast Chasm	231
48. Who Cares For ME? A Universal Care Approach to Myalgic Encephalomyelitis (ME)	234
49. Introduction to Essential Notes On How To Care	242
50. Essential Notes on How to Care by Alem Matthees and Helen Donovan	244
51. Attitudes	246
52. Saint or Sinner? Caring full time for someone diagnosed as having Very Severe ME	248
53. Partnership	253
54. What Wrong Assumptions Can You Easily Make	257
55. Carer Skills	262
56. A Mind/Body/Emotion/Spirit Approach	271
57. Do No Harm	274
58. How To Approach Someone With Severe or Very Severe ME: A Quick Check List	277
59. How To Help The Person With Severe or Very Severe ME	278
60. What does Being Present Actually mean, for People with Complex Symptom Experience and Hypersensitivity?	281
61. Presence Experienced as Physical Touch, by Christine Fenton	284
62. Caring for Someone Diagnosed with Severe or Very Severe ME, the Need to be Strong	285
63. A Quick Alphabet Of Points For Carers	288
64. A Wish For Carers	299
65. Self-Reflective Questions for Home Carers	300
66. Part Four: Communication Issues	307
67. Communication: a Complex issue	308
68. Blocks to Interaction	313
69. When You are Fearful	319
70. Active listening	321
71. Successful Listening	323
72. How To Listen To Each Other	331

73. How You might Approach Communication With Someone Unable To Directly Speak To You	333
74. Part Five: Impact Upon Relationships	337
75. Introduction to Verses From Invisible Octopus Poem by Corina Duyn	338
76. Verses from Invisible Octopus Poem by Corina Duyn	339
77. A Moment In Time	341
78. On being a Partner to Someone with Very Severe Chronic Illness	342
79. You Find a Way	346
80. Severe and Very Severe ME: the Unexpected Losses	347
81. The Poverty of Severe and Very Severe ME	354
82. Seven Useful Habits To Develop When You Live With Someone Diagnosed With Severe/Very Severe ME	357
83. Learning to Live in Smaller Spaces	364
84. Be the Change You Want to See	368
85. Part Six : Professional Input	370
86. Introduction to "Door Poster" by Soph Clark	371
87. A Door Poster by Soph Clark	372
88. Risk Assessment in Severe and Very Severe ME	374
89. Reasons why it is inappropriate to offer Cognitive Behaviour Therapy to someone diagnosed with Severe or Very Severe ME	379
90. The Core Components of a Proper ME service	384
91. Training For People Who Have to Engage With a Person Diagnosed with Severe or Very Severe ME in a Caring Capacity	392
92. Dentistry Issues	397
93. Acting as an Advocate	400
94. Not a patient For The Inexperienced Carer, by Wendy Boutilier (Global Advocates 4 ME-ICC)	402
95. Some Questions Worth Considering For Nurses and Others Offering Care	404
96. Self-Reflective Questions for Professionals Involved in Caring	408

97. Part Seven: Remembering Those Who Have Died	412
98. Severe Myalgic Encephalomyelitis, Understanding and Remembrance day, August 8th: Yes We Will Remember	413
99. Don't Let Us Down!	415
100. We Remember: a Reflection for Severe ME Day	421
101. A Trail of Love	423
102. A thank you to a friend who is dying	425
For More Information	427
Afterword	429
About the Author	431

1

OVERVIEW

> Until Severity and difference of severity experience is understood and fully recognised, services and healthcare will still not understand the real needs of people with Very Severe ME.'

Linda Crowhurst

∼

THIS BOOK, A SELECTION of Stonebird Guides and new writings gives you an overview of how you might approach relationship, interaction and care for people diagnosed with Severe/Very Severe ME with flexibility and compassion.

When faced with severe illness and complex symptom reaction, it is not easy to know how to respond appropriately, without triggering symptom deterioration. Whether in the context of decades of suffering or newly faced with the unexpected decline of a loved one into severe illness, it is not always obvious what to do and when to do it, in the best way. Time, patience, experience and an openness to learn the best way to support someone can help unimaginably. Honesty and sharing can help tremendously too.

It is equally not easy, for the person living with often invisible torment and complex symptom reaction, to get their needs safely met. The simplest ordinary thing, like a cough, sneeze, footstep, the sound of a knife on a plate or a movement in the room, can, for some, trigger a massive, unexpected reaction.

With communication difficulties ranging from slow to impossible and with variable and maybe profound environmental hypersensitivities, it can be very difficult to help the person in the best possible way, without unintentionally triggering an intolerable exacerbation.

This is why we have tried to raise awareness, over decades, of the symptoms, risks and difficulties in caring for those most severely ill, misunderstood, neglected and vulnerable.

And this is why we have developed the MOMENT approach to caring; a person-centred, partnership approach to offering care, which is based upon our own experience of trying to meet need in extremely difficult circumstances, with profound hypersensitivity, repeated paralysis and other, not easily understood, agonising symptom experience.

2

INTRODUCTION MOIRA DILLON FROM ME ADVOCATES IRELAND (MEAI)

～

We are fortunate to have access to so much of Greg and Linda's immensely helpful advice and notes on Severe/Very Severe ME. Greg's 'Notes For Carers'[1] provided simple, practical solutions to the everyday problems family and agency carers can face when looking after a person with Severe/Very Severe ME. More 'Notes for Carers' takes this further.

People with Severe/Very Severe ME experience substantial limitations, impairment, and disability - their symptom burden is great, and quality of life is poor. Most people with Severe/Very Severe ME are housebound and bedbound; some lie immobile for days. Some experience full body paralysis. The impaired physical functioning of those people with Severe/Very Severe ME may explain the difficulties individuals within the severe category of ME have accessing daily care. These factors must be considered when planning care routines and methods of engaging with such a fragile group.

It is so important to learn how to care for people with Severe/Very Severe ME and to be equipped to advise others on how best to care for those who are so frail and chronically ill. The purpose of Greg's notes is to disseminate the importance of what can and should be done for this hidden patient population. By focusing on the severely affected, it is Greg's hope that the morbid physiological nature of the disease will be better accepted and understood, and effective methods of patient care carried out. These invaluable notes will carefully guide and assist the carers of people with Severe /Very Severe ME to accomplish that.

I find that I keep going back to Greg's accounts of his experience of Severe/Very Severe ME and all his excellent care notes despite my collecting truly relevant feedback from patients with Severe/Very Severe ME, and from others who care for them. I have not come across anything else close to the high standard and quality of the records of first-hand experience of the incredibly serious nature of Severe/Very Severe ME through Greg's care for his wife Linda. For me, as a patient and advocate Greg's notes highlight an aspect of Severe/Very Severe ME I had been unaware of, the serious and severe physical illness underlying the person's symptom experience, and the importance of caring with great care to avoid harm.

Caring for people with ME at the severe end of the spectrum, can be extremely challenging to get right. A high level of carer skill and awareness is required because of the frailty of someone with Severe/Very Severe ME. People this ill are extremely vulnerable to harm through the wrong care approach. What the carer learns from Greg's notes will subtly impact on how caring is provided and will inevitably have a positive effect on the relationship, the quality of care and the health of the person receiving the care.

In his carers notes Greg offers a unique perspective into life as a carer to a loved one, exploring the love, the fears and the isolation experienced daily by a carer. Looking after a person with Severe/Very Severe ME can often leave carers emotionally and physically exhausted. Carers are particularly vulnerable to feeling stressed, worried, and run down by the vast demands that often come with caregiving.

This comprehensive, objective, and practical guide offers valuable advice on how carers can care for the patient and how best carers can care for themselves by doing the caring in the best, most appropriate ways possible. This is the book that should be given to carers when there is a diagnosis of Severe/Very Severe ME. Greg's notes should be essential reading for all carers of those with ME and for the families and friends of those suffering.

'More Notes for Carers', which builds on Greg's previous book, 'Notes For Carers' is an accessible and detailed guide which includes practical tips, checklists for best practice, descriptions of experience from a wide range of carers, practical advice that addresses solutions to common problems, and expert advice on how to deliver compassionate and dignified care to people with Severe/Very Severe ME. 'More Notes For Carers' is a comprehensive look at all caring and management aspects of Severe/Very Severe ME - physical, mental and emotional.

---

[1]. Notes For Carers, an illustrated handbook packed full of practical tips, insights, guides and exercises, is available at https://stonebird.co.uk/Notes/index.html

3
VALUABLE RESOURCES BY COLLEEN STECKEL, ME PATIENT AND ADVOCATE

MYALGIC ENCEPHALOMYELITIS IS A devastating disabling disease too often misunderstood as something that can be self managed without specialised care. ME patients have one of the lowest quality of life scores and yet often receive minimal medical support. Caregivers are often left mostly on their own, struggling to manage the needs of their severely ill loved ones.

Stonebird materials and the books put out by Greg Crowhurst have been valuable resources which I have shared often for many years.

Some of the information about paralysis in ME and the challenges of the most severely ill are seldom covered by others.

Greg's work has been instrumental in making sure this information has reached the community and medical health professionals.

Without his efforts, I am sure many more sufferers would

have been harmed due to lack of proper understanding and lack of proper care. As a 30+ year ME patient and long time advocate, when someone is asking me about Severe ME one of the first resources I recommend is Greg Crowhurst and his Stonebird website. I know many share my gratitude for all the work he has done providing guidance on being a caring caregiver.

FOREWORD BY GREG CROWHURST

~

BETWEEN US, MY WIFE and I have almost 55 years experience of living with Severe, then Very Severe ME. That gives us, I believe, a unique perspective, especially given that before ME struck my wife was a qualified Social Worker and Counsellor and I a qualified Nurse and Educator, both of us deeply committed and experienced in working in partnership with people who had a profound disability.

In this situation, you can never afford not to keep learning, growing, developing, in order to figure out the best way through each tortuous moment.

We have learned a great deal.

There is much to share. Compiling this book, under the circumstances, has been impossibly difficult; it will be my last on how to care for people diagnosed with Severe and Very Severe ME.

Like all the others, it is produced at great personal cost, in the midst of caring for someone with severe illness, profound, multiple disabilities, excruciating pain and paralysis so terrible that entire days and weeks can be lost by a sudden noise, a wrong movement or a misplaced question.

If there are any errors in layout or typography, all I can do is ask for your forgiveness. I can do no more, not at this stage.

Today, for example, as I write this, my wife woke me at 4am, saying that there was no part of her body that was not in great pain. She could not sleep. No position offered any comfort or rest. It is but a moment in an ocean of moments, where the suffering is overwhelming and the need painfully hard to meet.

If there are any major issues relating to the material, let me know and they hopefully can be dealt with in subsequent revisions.

Inevitably, in a manual like this, there is going to be some overlap and repetition. Some of the content has been previously published, some is new. The purpose is to gather together our most important material into one, easily accessible place.

For there is no guarantee that Stonebird, my website, will always exist. The book will be a separate resource, not just for those new to caring but also for those who may want to reflect deeper on their role.

As with my previous book, "Notes For Carers", this is a shared experience. I am proud to include insightful contributions from all around the world. I am particularly grateful to Linda, my wife, for sharing her experience, especially through her poetry.

The subject matter ranges from how to be present in the face of profound suffering, how to communicate effectively, how to listen, how to provide skilled care, all within the context of a person-centred, partnership approach to caring and relationship.

Perhaps because so much time has passed, decades of enduring the unimaginable, I find I need a book, exactly like this, myself. I need it to keep me focused, to remind me what is important, to renew my commitment to love and partnership.

I hope it helps you too.

PART ONE: THE SEVERE/VERY SEVERE ME EXPERIENCE

Welcome to Part One! Severe ME is a tormenting experience while Very Severe ME is a tortured, extreme existence, where nothing is possible and every single interaction is intense, deteriorative and intolerable.

Here we consider what it is like to live in those broken places of Severe/Very Severe ME.

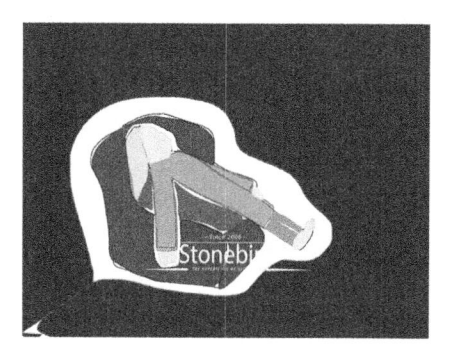

There are many different ways a person diagnosed with Severe or Very Severe ME can be neglected.

BROKEN PLACES

We live in the broken places
Very few know or comprehend.
We live on the edge of life,
Not knowing if or when we will fall off,
Yet clinging on,
Regardless of the intense, unbearable,
Indescribable levels
Of suffering.
We hold on to all that is good,
All that is true,
All that is life
And will ourselves onward
Towards hope that seems hopeless,
Yet still we demand of it
To come to our aid.
In spite of the unlikeliness,
We trust in tomorrow,
Even when today is tortured,

Unbearable,
Impossible even,
Yet we do not give in to despair.
Despite our own agony
Or even, because of it,
Because we know what most cannot even glimpse,
We hold out invisible hands
And create a network of love
To gently embrace, surround and comfort
Those in desperate need.
In the void of clinical neglect
And abject torment,
We will each other on
Where the world has turned its back
And simply has no answers,
Nor recognition
As a result.
We somehow endure
And be
The bedrock
Of missing support,
Laced together by love,
Reaching out towards the gap between heartbeats,
Praying and asking that
We survive another day.

7

THE DISEASE MYALGIC ENCEPHALOMYELITIS

~

UNFORTUNATELY THE DISEASE MYALGIC Encephalomyelitis [1] has been buried in the generalised terms of ME/CFS, CFS/ME, CFS or Chronic Fatigue.

Myalgic Encephalomyelitis[2] surely must be unique among diseases in how, in the absence of a test or clearly defined diagnostic criteria, it is driven more by what any individual believes it to be or by what any vested interest promotes it to be.

There is no one specific clear clinical picture used to reassure patients and confirm diagnosis. [3] The biopsychosocial expansion of the term "ME" to mean something quite different to the original Enteroviral Disease[4], coined by Ramsay[5], means that no one can really know what disease they have and whether it is treatable or not.

Nowadays it seems to us that the causative factors are ignored and the underlying physiology, in relation to the specific symptoms that people are experiencing, is not identified or explained adequately.

Without this core information ME is alarmingly wide open to be misinterpreted as a mental health issue, as can be witnessed, world wide, across Health Service provision.

These days we are much more comfortable using the term "diagnosed with Severe ME". This is because nobody can tell for sure who has Myalgic Encephalomyelitis, not unless they had a VP1 Test, which was abandoned in the UK in the 1980's [6].

It is important to recognise that there are different categories of Severity: Mild, Moderate, Severe and Very Severe: increasingly it is clear to us that a clear separation between the categories of "Severe" and "Very Severe" ME is necessary to protect the most ill.

According to the ME Association, only 2% of people will have Very Severe ME. (Flemming 2017). Our focus on Stonebird is firmly towards the two percent, because that is our fundamental experience.

In Very Severe ME the depth of suffering is unimaginable until experienced. It is a tortured, extreme existence, where nothing is possible and every single interaction is intense, deteriorative and intolerable.

It cannot be emphasised enough that it is a devastating, life changing illness of vast proportion with unquantifiable impact. Here it can feel like death is often imminent and life is unsustainable.

Current criteria understate the range of hypersensitivities and other symptoms that can completely incapacitate and isolate or alienate and utterly disable a person, long term.

Severe/Very Severe ME impacts all levels of life and relationships in ways that cannot necessarily be described fully.

There may be difficulties in gaining access to physical care, benefits, medical investigations and appropriate long-term medical support.

One is always aware that for the most severely ill, the risk of death from ME or in some cases from other undiagnosed comorbid conditions, is a very real possibility.

There is also the tragic loss of life from suicide that too often results from a lack of medical understanding. Each person's death is felt painfully by the ME community.

The seriousness of this disease and the pathology of the disease is hard to prove. Yet, when demonstrated, for example, through post-mortem, Dorsal Root Ganglionitis[7] and inflammation, it shows the off the scale suffering which people with Severe/Very ME endure.

There is a great need to recognise the range of symptoms, such as muscle spasm, paralysis, the severity of cognitive dysfunction and the complex hypersensitivities, as well as Post-Exertional Malaise (PEM) or Post Exertional Neuro-immune Exhaustion (PENE), the more recent, preferred term.

It is so necessary not to clinicalise these words or detach them from the terrible reality that the person experiences, moment by moment.

Within the "Severe" category, there may be differences of ability, some people may be able to move sporadically, whereas for others the slightest exertion such as thinking, trying to speak, remembering or attempting any sort of two-way interaction can trigger PENE or longer deterioration. Each person is different.

It is important to try and understand that what the ordinary person recognises as exertion is way beyond the capacity of someone diagnosed with Severe or Very Severe ME. Any exertion at all, on any level, however tiny or minimal or not even noticeable to the untrained eye, can still have a deteriorative impact leading to a worsening of symptoms, short or long term.

Pain and other symptoms may be so extreme that being touched or lifted might be completely intolerable.

That may be hard to understand and challenging to learn.

> Carers may be confronted with very frightening symptoms and not know what to do or the best way to interact or help without risking triggering deterioration. Professionals may also have no more of a clue as to how to proceed than anyone else.

People with Very Severe ME experience intense, never-ending suffering. Some may be exceedingly weak, however others will actually experience muscle paralysis. It can be very frightening, especially if new to this level of symptom experience, to observe and it will not necessarily be obvious as to the best way to help them.

When a person is paralysed, for example, the carer may think that they are just resting or asleep, when in fact they may be desperate for help, thirsty, too cold, too hot, in intolerable pain, screaming agony, too blank to think, too paralysed to speak or open their eyes.

The carer may also be confronted with the possibility or fear that the person has died, especially when breathing is extremely shallow and no movement is visible. That is a very real scenario for those caring for the most severely ill.

Each person will have their own unique experience of ME, depending on their specific combination and interaction of symptoms and the underlying physiology of those symptoms. Not enough is known about this.

Difficulty with swallowing, chewing, choking, severe food

sensitivities and gastric issues may all be found in the most ill, to varying degrees.

There is a great need for proper medical support for all people with ME, but especially for those with complex symptom experience. However there can be great difficulty getting good GP input and right response.

Very ill people certainly do not need to be arguing how severely disabled they are, because of a lack of medical understanding and recognition.

GP's need to take long-term responsibility for their patients.

The doctor needs to recognise that ME is a WHO neurological disease with multi-system dysfunction, rather than a mental health fatigue condition, which should elicit a completely different response.

Prognosis is an important issue. There is a big difference in the prognosis between children/ young adults and older adults. [8]The prognosis is poor for older adults who have not shown significant improvement within five years of being ill.

[9] A realistic representation of prognosis is essential in order to help people understand the nature of their illness and how to adapt to it.

This is not a short term illness, rather it is a complex, difficult to bear physical disease that lasts for many years and decades.

Ongoing support demands highly skilled care, that is what we are going to look at now.

---

1. This article is extracted and expanded from our review of a series of films on Severe ME called *Dialogues*. The full review can be read here: https://stonebird.co.uk/dialogues/index.html
2. The term Myalgic Encephalomyelitis (ME) was first used in an anonymous editorial in an issue of the Lancet. (Jason et al 2014 **Are Myalgic**

Encephalomyelitis and chronic fatigue syndrome different illnesses? A preliminary analysis https://www.ncbi.nlm.nih.gov/pmc/articles/PMC4125561/#R1

3. According to Dr Byron Hyde, the term "CFS"represents well over 100 pathologies or diseases.
4. Enteroviruses were the original pathogen suspected to cause ME.

    Enteroviruses are responsible for a wide variety of human diseases ranging from mild gastroenteritis to full multi-organ failure. Comprised of Polioviruses, Coxsackieviruses A&B, Echoviruses and E71, the enterovirus genus is a member of the Picornaviridea family marked by its extremely small size.

    While Poliomyelitis has virtually been eradicated in the Western world, others of the genera have filled the vacuum so created. Enteroviruses, remarkably resistant to its harsh conditions, persist in the gut.
5. For background information on the history of ME, please see GAME: https://artzstudios1.wixsite.com/globaladvocatesmeicc/portfolio
6. For more information on the VP1 test please see : http://carersfight.blogspot.com/2016/05/why-separation-of-me-from-cfs-is-long.html
7. The coroner's verdict in 2006 that Sophia Mirza's spinal cord showed inflammation caused by dorsal root ganglionitis , was a major breakthrough for the ME Community. In 2018 Merryn Croft's post mortem showed inflammation of the ganglia.
8. See the ME Association: **Children and Adolescents** https://meassociation.org.uk/about-what-is-mecfs/children-and-adolescents/
9. The US Centers for Disease Control (CDC) cited a review of published studies reporting recovery rates of 8–63% (median 40%), with full recovery being rare (5–10% achieving total remission). https://www.ncbi.nlm.nih.gov/books/NBK53583/

8
PEOPLE

People of the world look
but see us not
Listen,
but hear us not
Speak,
but miss the point.
Instead we turn to each other......

9
BARRIERS TO CONNECTION

∽

There are many barriers to connection that are not obvious to the well person, that create broken interactions and impossibilities, in many if not most or all moments.

- Internal body level
- External body level
- Immediate environment level
- Wider environment level
- Medical Misinformation level
- Social level
- Political level

Each level adds a further layer of barrier between the person, the world and you.

Each barrier described below is a layer of isolation from normality. Add them all together and you have a thick wall of barrier after barrier, that creates an exclusion from normality and a necessity to live separately to survive.

The isolation and sense of alienation is profound.

Internal body level

Internally there is much going on that is fragmenting, painful and empty.

Cognitive dysfunction can be extreme and under represented in terms of its devastating reality.

It may take time to kick in and become apparent or worsen significantly.

A person may struggle with finding words, familiar names, putting names to faces, speaking words oddly, with letters switched round for an individual word or mixed between words so that eg red strawberry will become "straw redberry". Or a wrong word will be used, like intending to say I want a sandwich but instead saying I want "a machine" or some other totally unrelated word.

Vocabulary may be minimised at times so that expression is limited. In worst case scenarios the mind may be completely blanked out, short term memory forgotten, words may be inaccessible, thoughts may be gone, visualisation may be lost, incoming information may be totally overloading or overstimulating and literally physically painful to try and understand.

One-way communication may be all that is tolerable or possible. Ideas may float into view then disappear the next before they can be grasped and expressed.

Sometimes sentences remain half finished as the mind blanks out the rest of what was intended to be spoken.

If their ability to communicate varies and the person only has contact when it might be possible to think a little, then the true reality of their cognitive difficulties may be denied by others, downplayed, dismissed, laughed off, misunderstood, which leads the person, who is struggling to relate, even more invalidated and isolated.

> Even at best the possibility of expression may be limited and far less than before the person was ill.

The speed at which you speak is very important, as words can become meaningless strings of noise, if uttered too quickly or for too long. Processing may be very slow, delayed or impossibly hard, in any given moment.

Pain is a massive invisible barrier that at its worst takes all the person's time, attention and focus to endure, leaving no energy or ability to even tolerate another's presence in the room. Some sorts of pain may be more extreme or intolerable than others. This sort of pain is hard to impossible to get under control, yet again, may not be fully recognised by others especially if they have had no experience of severe disabling pain themselves.

> For those with the most severe constant, high level pain, untreatable, unmanageable by medicine, life must be taken moment by moment in excruciating agony.

The way pain is experienced can feel like a further barrier still, in that normally rest would be expected to brings relief, restoration, healing, comfort, but for the person whose pain only increases with stillness and rest, whose pain only intensifies and varies in the immensity of pain, with various shifting regions of the body, alongside varying different forms of pain, such as burning, throbbing, itching, crawling, stabbing pain.

How unhelpful it is to that person to be told by other well-meaning folk to 'rest and feel better soon'. It is just never going to happen and adds to the very real burden of denial, downplaying and isolation that a person can feel.

Muscle fatigue and muscle weakness can feel completely overwhelming and indescribably assaulting in its own, unique, emptying way.

Lack of energy makes it exhausting to think, let alone move or try to interact or do anything with or without help.

The experience of everything and everyone, being completely out of reach, can feel inexplicable, can create a sense of an invisible wall around you that you cannot breach in any way, yet which no one else can see around you or understand how tangible and physically limiting it is.

Noise sensitivity is a massive barrier to connecting. It is both an internal hazard and an external one. It hits you both internally and externally, with the vibration.

It is important that anyone who tries to communicate with a person with noise sensitivity understand what they might need to do in order to make the interaction tolerable, bearable or possible. Without awareness, a voice too loud can cause unimaginable pain, disorientation, suffering, that may continue long after the seemingly small, too loud sentence has been uttered, but which is completely invisible.

Though there may be visible symptoms triggered by the noise such as muscle spasm, crying out; the internal havoc noise wreaks is impossibly hard to describe in the most severely affected, creating a severe shut down of body and mind.

You need to understand how you impact the person, even if you do not fully understand or comprehend the person's inner experience. Every movement makes noise. Every noise can batter, hurt, confuse. This is probably way beyond the understanding of most people. It creates a wall of separation and isolation, especially if it is not totally accepted and adapted to as much as is possible.

The need to avoid noise in order to protect yourself, from very real physical harm, from sound that has no apparent affect on any one else, can look or feel bizarre, extreme and odd or be misinterpreted as anti-social or exaggerating. The torment of invisibility and misinterpretation is itself, then, a painful barrier.

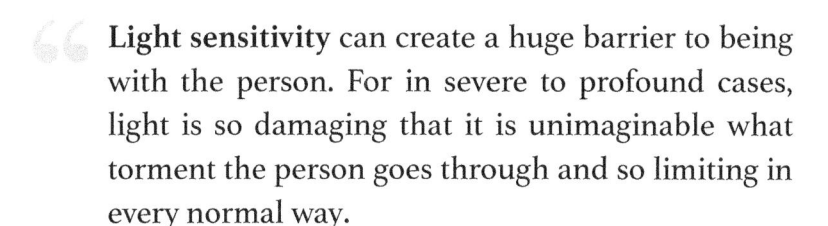

> **Light sensitivity** can create a huge barrier to being with the person. For in severe to profound cases, light is so damaging that it is unimaginable what torment the person goes through and so limiting in every normal way.

Texting, phoning, using a computer, watching TV, turning a light casually on, experiencing ordinary levels of sunlight or even dull day light, can have a profound, painful affect.

Every social contact or carer contact, every medical intervention, will be affected by this symptom and impact the way interaction can occur safely. This can be a huge barrier to try to overcome, in order to maintain any shared interaction safely, comfortably or at all and get needs met.

Numbness may be widespread and constant or variable in degree.

The person who experiences numb limbs or other parts of the body is already separated from normal sensation and feeling. The environment can then become dangerous if this means the person can not safely tell temperature, can lead to burns from wrongly assessing the heat of something.

Not only this, proprioception can be lost impacting spacial orientation and awareness. There is so often a loss of recognition that the symptoms are either real or have potentially serious implications if not recognised or acknowledged.

To say the word "numbness" does not convey the ongoing internal experience of not feeling your body, not feeling your environment, not being able to safely judge with touch, what things feel like or if you are wet or hot or cold or safe or developing a pressure sore.

To not be able to feel the tenderness of a touch, but to have it distorted instead, by numbness, without even considering the additional issues that pain, severe pins and needles and hyperesthesia might bring, can be devastating.

This can bring up barriers to intimacy, barriers to providing or getting safe care.

Yet numbness can vary in intensity and is extremely important to recognise. Without this, it just becomes a further barrier between the experience of the person and being seen for their true reality. It can lead to further alienation and an even wider layer of isolation from others.

Paralysis is a much neglected symptom of ME. It is not included in later diagnostic criteria despite the early medical founders acknowledging it and there is a well-defined potential association, through Enterovirus to Polio and paralysis, that makes great sense.

Trying to get safe and accurate diagnosis and support for

this symptom is fraught with difficulty, not least because of the risk of psychiatric misdiagnosis as FND, Functional Neurological Disorder and the danger that underlying pathology will be ignored or not sought adequately. This is not helped by the lack of medical interest in paralysis in ME.

Without understanding the pathology, there is risk of mistreatment and misinterpretation. This leads to the neglect of the most ill, who have the most difficulty in accessing services, tolerating investigation, gaining access to the right medical consultants or getting needs met.

Not only is there the barrier of **denial and medical neglect**, there can then also be the denial, downplaying or misunderstanding that paralysis receives from society, social contacts and family, as well as the extremely painful and difficult reality itself, of being repeatedly or long term paralysed, which can impact every level of existence.

The isolation on a physical level is huge for the person who is continually paralysed and unable to speak or move or partially paralysed. The after impact can be equally devastating in its own way, taking many hours or days to throw it off, partially, if at all. The blocks to doing anything by yourself, for yourself, even if help is available or even being with anyone else, are vast and huge and indescribable. The desperate need for input that never comes is tragic.

> The lack of kindness or recognition is demolishing.
> The lack of empathy is staggering.

The vast void between the ordinary life and the person invisibly experiencing paralysis, with an ME diagnosis, as opposed to any other disease where it is medically respected and honoured, is the difference between a proper service and medical neglect and complete separation from kindness and validation.

External body level

Hyperesthesia, an inability to tolerate light touch, makes a huge barrier to intimacy, affection and meeting even basic care needs. Contact that might have felt previously pleasurable, before ill health came, may becomes a tormenting experience instead.

A gentle touch may feel like a sledge hammer blow, a comforting stroke on the arm might receive the sort of reaction equivalent that which you might get from someone irritated by nails scratching down a blackboard; intolerable, screamingly unbearable, not in keeping with the gentleness and kindness or warmth a person might have hoped to convey.

If the person flinches on the slightest contact, how can more wanted, intimate moments be achieved? The barrier to tender intimacy is vast. It is difficult in these circumstances to offer any of the usual ways of physically expressing genuine affection.

The barrier to get any physically help is also problematic.

- How do you lift someone who cannot bear contact on their skin?
- How can you wear comfortable clothes that you feel good in, if material on your skin irritates, hurts, feels as if it is you crushing you?
- How can you protect your feet or find suitable footwear when any pressure on your feet is agony?
- How can you keep warm in bed if the lightest sheet over you hurts you?
- How can you cover your eyes to protect yourself from light, if you cannot tolerate sunglasses on your nose or eye masks on your face?

- How can you protect against torturing sound, if you cannot put earplugs in your ears, due to the pain of pressure in your ears or wear ear defenders on your ears or cope with the pressure on your head, due to hyperesthesia?
- How can you get back or neck support to help you sit up supported, if you cannot tolerate touch or pressure?
- How can you lie in bed when the pillow pressure causes massive pain against your head?
- And how does the person, who simply does not fit neatly into any regular system, because they do not have the standard average, usual, general issues that people experience, in the same standard way, actually get their complex needs recognised or met?

There are no easy answers. As with most aspects of this disabling diagnosis, there is little understanding, few appropriate aids that are geared to the specific challenges faced by people with severe hypersensitivity, that arise and leave the person feeling even more alienated by a system that does not provide for them adequately or even recognise the tormented state that they are left in.

Movement sensitivity is incredibly disabling.

- How can a person easily be with anyone else if every movement they make affects them painfully? This instantly creates a barrier between people. If any movement is a threat to your health, it is incredibly hard to feel safe around other people. At worst it can trigger muscle spasm, muscle paralysis, weakness,

shock, disorientation, intensified pain and other worsening of symptoms.
- How can you use a wheelchair then, if you are not able to be mobile without one or only minimally so, but cannot bear the sensation of motion or things or people moving near or past you?
- How can you share a conversation with someone else, if the risk of them moving their hand, tapping their foot, gesticulating wildly, without awareness, can harm you, confuse you, shut your mind down, increase your pain, nausea, headache, drain your energy?

> What unimaginably complex barriers do people with movement hypersensitivity have to endure? What sense of isolation and separation must they experience? Indescribable.

Chemical/perfume sensitivity is an invisible major barrier. It impacts most areas of living. It is almost impossible to completely protect yourself from exposure, people carry it on their clothing, their accessories, their coats, their hands, their hair.

At best, the smell is unpleasant, at worst it can trigger severe reactions.

It is hard to get people to take it seriously or to understand quite how badly they affect you. They smell perfume less on themselves as they get used to it. People are not necessarily willing to change their ways enough to make a difference.

> How many are willing to use fragrance free, perfume-free products, not just on the day they

visit, but regularly so it is not stuck to hair, clothing, handbags, hats etc.? It is not just about not using perfumed soap, it requires discipline to not use a perfumed product to wash your hair, for personal hygiene, to clean your house, to do your washing.

If you wear clean clothes but then sit on a car seat full of perfume, because you normally wear it or the person driving you wears it all the time or you have to use public transport or you handle money and get it on your hands, all the other effort, if you have made it is wasted.

Perhaps your pet uses flea treatment or has perfume on its coat? You are still carrying perfume or chemicals on you that could negatively impact the vulnerable person who has MCS.

It is not easy. It takes a huge commitment to understand and recognise the need of the other person and commit to the removal of all products in your own life that might affect them.

Otherwise letters parcels, gifts all become unwanted perfume hazards.

A hug can range from unpleasant to down right dangerous, if you have throat paralysis as a consequence or breathing difficulties. It is an incredibly lonely experience to feel separated from everyone due to their lack or willingness to understand and take action to avoid contaminating you or your environment, to protect you from harm in order to maintain any semblance of contact or respect.

Other symptoms may vary for each person. Each person has their own particular mixture of symptoms, that can have an internal and/or external impact, that erects a barrier between them and everyone else.

Every single symptom creates its own unique barrier,

causing its own invisible suffering, building up layer upon layer of complex hurdles, for both the person and anyone who wants to be in their life, with them, however momentarily.

Immediate environmental level

The immediate environment can support the needs of the person or be an additional hostile problem. Any need that goes unmet is an extra layer of pain, exhaustion and potential for symptom deterioration.

It is very hard to create a safe environment, due to a range of issues:

Poverty prevents the affordability of items that might help ease the discomfort.

Lack of vision means that there is no special provision or understanding of the specific complex adaptations that people might need even to basic equipment. There are no special aids or equipment or clothing created or geared specially for hypersensitive people with ME, their issues ill thought through, nothing specifically available, to our knowledge, for this group of misinterpreted, misunderstood people, created to help them if they do not fit into standard provision.

> **Multiple Chemical Sensitivity** is a massive boundary to purchasing new household goods, getting even basics safely provided or accessing services others take for granted that can improve the environment, incase they trigger massive symptom reactions.

Level of severity of illness also impacts the quality of the environment.

If you cannot tolerate anyone in the room, it is hard to get it cleaned let alone redecorated, it is hard to get your bed made, let alone buy new beautiful furnishings, if it is impossible to tolerate light, colour, pattern, it is hard to have anything but the simplest plain decoration.

If you have visual and cognitive difficulties it may be impossibly difficult to tolerate or have beautiful things to look at, it can be difficult to look at anything at all.

If you are **sound sensitive**, it is impossible to tolerate the slightest help that you need, let alone make major changes to your home or room.

Wider environmental level

It is extremely hard to control your external environment, beyond asking people, if possible, to understand and respect your reality.

Complaint may or may not be effective. Living in an inappropriate environment can worsen and deteriorate health long term. It can create unpleasant to intolerable experiences.

The difference between having sensitive, kind, understanding people around you and deliberately ignorant people, is the difference between acceptance and feeling like a pariah in your own life.

Medical misinformation level

The barriers to safety and finding appropriate medical provision are unquantifiable.

> In a system that has neglected providing a biomedical pathway, despite decades of patient demand, it is impossibly hard to feel safe or genuinely understood.

All the time **physical pathology** is unknown, ignored, denied, all the time the cause of the disease is not sought, not acknowledged, misdirected away from, there will be no safe guidance or treatment.

The necessary understanding and truth of the disease will not be found and ME services will continue to fail people, especially the most ill.

Clinical diagnosis will continue, in effect, to be guesswork, based on poor criteria that do not specifically identify a disease, treatment will be hit and miss, as to whether it is safe or effective.

All the time research is done on a vague group of people, without identifying the cause, the information obtained will still be generalised and not clear enough to help get better diagnosis. And people's hope for better physiological recognition and understanding, treatment and cure are unlikely to be reliably met.

This leaves the most ill, often too ill to participate in research anyway, abandoned and misinterpreted.

Social level

There is great hurt when a person does not accept or believe your physical reality and interprets it as less than it is. The ice cold barrier of hurt, grows thicker and more impenetrable with each passing year.

The lack of understanding about the physical illness the person is experiencing can lead to misinterpretation and separation. People leave, others remain but ignore the truth, downplay it, miss a point of genuine connection, warmth and growth that might have been possible if only they were able or willing to convey recognition and comprehension.

> The fact that people do not appear to know why you are not physically in their lives, can be very upsetting.

The shocking insight that people may not be interested or apparently able to really even attempt to empathise with the terrible suffering that you are enduring, that never goes away, is an eye-opener. The broken pathways to communication can be demolishing and utterly negating.

There are continual losses that mount up. They may be impossible to deal with face to face or at all and there could be understandable grief with each new personal affront and ignorance that you experience from the hurt or harm caused by the ignorance of others, whether through disinterest, careless language, lack of understanding, denial of your reality, environmental assaults or abandonment.

The barriers to connection are vast, just from the sheer number of things that have been lost, yet which are ignored or forgotten or blamed upon you, as if you had somehow made a choice to be so ill that you could not see people or socialise.

The sense of invisibility, the very real isolation and feeling of inequality, mounts up continually, creating a higher and higher barrier to relationship-healing and connection.

Political level

Everything to do with ME has an underlying political agenda buried beneath it.

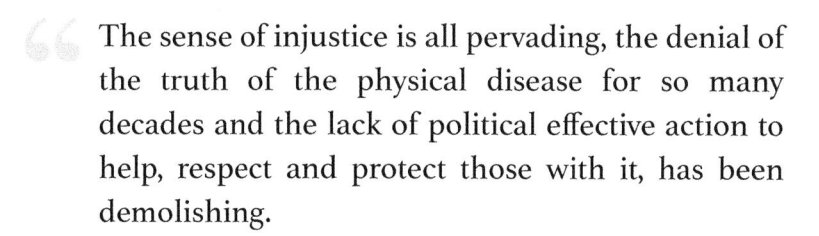

> The sense of injustice is all pervading, the denial of the truth of the physical disease for so many decades and the lack of political effective action to help, respect and protect those with it, has been demolishing.

This further builds a sense of isolation and negation, that there are those with genuine diseases who will be effectively provided for, recognised and supported but the disease ME is not one of them, as highlighted by the COVID Pandemic, for example.

The misinformation that has been allowed to continue in relation to this disease is shocking. The misinterpretation of the disease as a vague fatigue condition with no underlying pathology has been enabled to continue by ineffective political action over decades.

10

NEGLECT IN SEVERE AND VERY SEVERE ME

∼

Neglect can take on many forms. It leaves the person isolated, alienated, their needs unmet, harmed by inappropriate interventions or hurt by people's ignorance and carelessness.

There are many different ways a person diagnosed with Severe or Very Severe ME can be neglected.

The person may not be listened to.

If there are communication difficulties due to physical disability or cognitive dysfunction, it is very easy to not see, hear or notice need. The person may struggle to express, articulate or explain their need, which might be invisible, or because symptoms can fluctuate, an impression of greater ability than is actually present may be presented.

The person may be too ill to tolerate the presence of others, in order to get their needs met. Or the system might be too inflexible to provide in the right way for the person.

The person may articulate their need, yet still be dismissed or misinterpreted or misrepresented or misunderstood, if it does not fit in with the system's basic assumptions about them. If it is felt that all you need is encouragement or to push yourself, the person is particularly vulnerable to neglect.

The person may very well know what they want, but it might not be available, on offer or provided for 'ME', even if it is provided for people with other better recognised, acknowledged diseases.

Neglect is multi-faceted as there are so many ways that a person can be mistreated and their health or care needs not seen, recognised or met.

> If you do not understand or accept the limiting physical nature of the disease, the intense suffering a person is going through, the dangers of post-exertional deterioration, the need for support in all things, then there is a danger that you will either encourage the person to do more than is possible or safe or leave them without basic help, thinking they will do it themselves eventually.

A person may then not get the help that they need in the right way or maybe only get it partially met, even for the most basic things, such as help to eat, drink, cook, wash, take medicine or get to the toilet.

These are some things we have first hand experience of from other people over decades of severe disability and total high level care needs.

ATTITUDE: NOT BELIEVING THAT THE SYMPTOMS ARE REALLY BEING EXPERIENCED OR ARE THAT SEVERE.

RESPONSE: *'I don't believe you are in pain.'*

ATTITUDE: Denying particular symptoms altogether such as cognitive dysfunction.

RESPONSE: '*There is nothing wrong with your mind.*'

ATTITUDE: Not understanding or accepting the reality of severe illness.

RESPONSE: '*Get a life.*'

ATTITUDE: Not believing you need help.

RESPONSE: '*I know all you need is encouragement!*'

ATTITUDE: Not accepting a specific need for what it is, but instead arguing for something inappropriate, unusable and cheaper to provide.

RESPONSE: '*You can have a shower provided, not a bath.*'

ATTITUDE: Not offering help to get up off the bed whilst physically paralysed and unable.

RESPONSE: '*You can just push yourself up, 'I won't lift you*'

ATTITUDE: Not offering help to eat.

RESPONSE: '*You can eat this yourself*', *whilst totally paralysed and unable to speak or chew or move.*

ATTITUDE: Provision of wrong treatment regimes.

RESPONSE: '*We have tried it your way, now you must take Anti-depressants.*'

'*Unless you do what we say, you won't get well.*'

ATTITUDE: A lack of understanding of the severity of illness.

RESPONSE: '*Have a baby and get on with your life.*'

'*I expect you to come to the surgery.*'

'*What sort of service do you expect?*'

ATTITUDE: Denial of reality.

RESPONSE: '*Hope you are both well?*'

Not everything needs to be an overt, spoken insult that leads to denial. Often it is more subtle than that, leaving the person negated, denied, not seen or heard.

It is hard to keep trying to explain your need to people and finding your need or request falls on deaf ears, like please don't wear perfume.

Or please don't send me perfumed gifts or make sure the perfume you wear does not get on any letter or card or clothes or present.

Or please do not give me food or sweets that I cannot eat because many foods are unsuitable for me.

Or please do not ignore my symptoms, like noise sensitivity because they are an inconvenience to you.

Or please do not misinterpret my inability as choice.

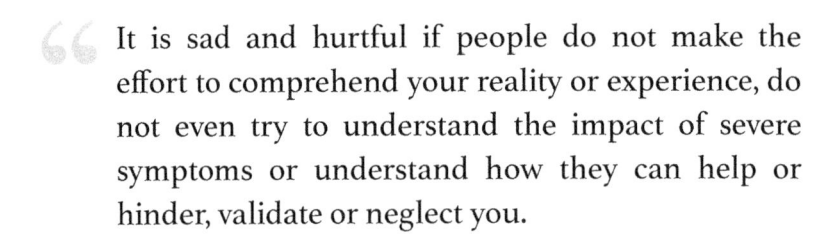

> It is sad and hurtful if people do not make the effort to comprehend your reality or experience, do not even try to understand the impact of severe symptoms or understand how they can help or hinder, validate or neglect you.

What does neglect look like?

- Invisibility
- Not provided for
- Medical, social, care needs not met
- Drugs not put out
- Food not in reach
- Equipment and suitable aids not provided
- Ignorance
- Professional superiority
- Arrogance
- Patronising
- One-sided opinion
- Self-importance

- Misinterpretation
- Misrepresentation
- Denial
- Sarcasm
- Mistreatment
- No treatment
- Ignoring vital signs
- Self-righteousness
- Judgment
- Limits
- Blame
- Harm
- Deterioration
- Abandonment
- Wrong assumptions
- Lies
- Misreporting
- Defensive justification

What does neglect feel like?

- Negation
- Disrespected
- Hurtful
- Lost
- Hopeless
- Helpless
- Angry
- Violated
- Judged
- Persecuted
- Denied

- Dismissed
- Ignored
- Not listened to
- Not heard
- Not interested in
- No compassion
- No empathy
- No recognition
- Not seen
- Not acknowledged
- Mistreated
- No treatment
- Blame
- Lack of accountability
- Pretence
- Loss
- Disconnected
- Alienated
- Misrepresented
- Misinterpreted
- Misinformed
- Omitted
- Uninvestigated
- Agony
- Insignificant
- Irrelevant
- Lonely
- Alone
- Estranged
- Negated
- Passed by
- Crushed

- Unequal
- Nothing
- Rejected
- Dismissed
- Refused
- Unimportant
- Worthless
- Afraid
- Unsafe
- Forsaken
- Uncared for
- Oppressed
- Invalid

What would negate neglect?

- Understanding
- Respect
- Acceptance
- Listening
- Taking right action
- Honesty
- Integrity
- Caring
- Reaching out
- Acknowledging
- Trying to get things right
- Effort
- Compassion
- Empathy
- Attention
- Detail

- Understanding symptom impact
- Recognising the effect of symptoms
- Patience
- Affirmation
- Genuineness
- Humility
- Desire to truly help
- Changing habits
- Growing together
- Connection
- Communication
- Partnership
- Understanding
- Valuing
- Apology
- Consideration
- Intention
- Acknowledgment
- Advocacy

11

THE PARADOX OF CARING FOR PEOPLE DIAGNOSED WITH SEVERE OR VERY SEVERE ME

∽

THERE ARE PARADOXES THAT may only become apparent when you try to engage with and care for people diagnosed with Severe /Very Severe ME.

It is not necessarily obvious as to how and when to interact safely with the person and in the best way. This book advocates a person-centred, moment-centred, moment aware posture and approach to care.

People with Severe ME are roughly 25% of the ME population. People with Severe ME are roughly 2% [1] of the ME population. For them, it seems, there is little comprehension of what they go through or how to safely help and interact with them. Some will be more able than others, in very limited ways.

People's experience may vary from day to day and moment to moment but always in the context of severe illness and multi-system dysfunction. For some there is no let up to the high intensity of their symptoms. Their needs are complex. There are a number of paradoxes that may only become apparent when you try to engage with the person.

I need help, but.... there is always a but.

Receiving care is not easy, straightforward nor is it necessarily obvious, as to how and when to interact safely and in the best way for the person.

Everyone experiences their symptoms uniquely, yet there will be common experiences and common difficulties in accessing care.

I personally never found painkillers that alleviated my pain. Neither could I tolerate them. The pain of Very Severe ME is unquenchable and intense. The symptom experience is unimaginable to those who have never known it, the level of tormenting hypersensitivities to ordinary things indescribably disturbing and assaulting, adding to the difficulty of getting safe and supportive, experienced care.

I need physical care but.... I cannot tolerate physical contact, because of a range of symptoms that directly affect how I experience and tolerate anyone's presence in the room or physically helping me:

- Hyperesthesia
- Pressure intolerance
- Severe pain
- Noise sensitivity
- Light sensitivity
- Headache
- Confusion
- Disorientation
- No energy
- Sleep difficulties
- Touch sensitivity

- Perfume/ chemical sensitivity
- Cognitive dysfunction
- Chewing, swallowing difficulties
- Movement sensitivity
- Motion sensitivity
- Muscle spasms
- Breathlessness
- Periodic paralysis
- Muscle weakness
- Muscle fatigue
- Post-exertional exacerbation of symptoms

I experience all these symptoms every day severely, yet some are more intense than others and some may vary in intensity through the day and night. I am in a continual state of moving toward, away or stuck in paralysis, that makes engagement with others virtually impossible and extremely painful at best.

I experience hyperesthesia which means any contact, even if very light, is intolerable and extremely irritating. This makes clothing difficult to put on and wear, physical contact to try and help, even a kind gentle touch of reassurance is unpleasant and painfully irritating or for me, triggers paralysis if wrongly timed.

I cannot bear being stroked or massaged or comforted normally. I am always extremely touch sensitive and any touch may cause flinching, shaking, extreme pain, irritation, irritability, upset, mental confusion, disorientation, shock, paralysis, weakness, overstimulation, overwhelming exhaustion.

I experience severe pressure sensitivity making any physical pressure on my body anywhere intensify my pain, to the point that I might shout out if you do touch me or if you lean my body in such a way that there is increased pressure on any part of my body, especially my head, back or neck.

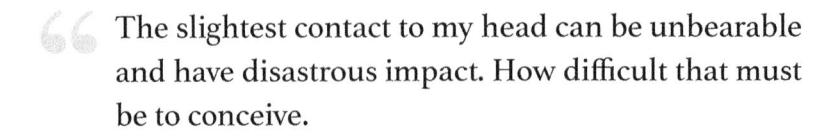

> The slightest contact to my head can be unbearable and have disastrous impact. How difficult that must be to conceive.

This means I cannot sit up with back or neck support, as contact on my neck or head cause intensifying pain. I am never comfortable. I cannot access the physical support I need, yet which will work against me if I get it. This is the strange, paradoxical life that you exist in with the worst level of hypersensitivities.

I always experience all over, severe to extreme pain. All my energy often goes into coping with the indescribable different sensations of pain: throbbing, burning, itching, crawling, shifting, stabbing. All this alongside terrible weakness and screamingly numb, empty feelings in my muscles.

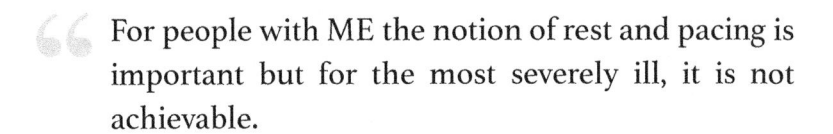

> For people with ME the notion of rest and pacing is important but for the most severely ill, it is not achievable.

For myself, rest, relaxation and sleep all lead to increasing weakness and paralysis. That is another paradox that the carer needs to understand. Everyone is different. All ordinary concepts such as 'rest helps you feel better' are turned on their head especially when it leads to continual paralysis or worsening weakness.

I have acute noise sensitivity. Every noise that you might make in the room is an assault upon me. It is literally a torture if it continues; even things that you may not be aware of or recognise as an issue, like clothes swishing, coughing, footsteps, doors shutting, scratching your head, are tormenting and painful at best.

Noise literally paralyses me, for hours on end, leaves me unable to move or even call out for help. My noise sensitivity is extreme, however try moving about the house and performing tasks without noise - it is virtually impossible. Yet when you need total silence to survive, that is absolutely what you need, not even someone doing things quietly, will do, no matter how hard they try.

I can be severely to extremely light sensitivity. Any exposure or any increased exposure to light can trigger intense burning, throbbing, eye pain and head pain, extremely painful after image, intense headache, mental anguish, confusion, disorientation, shock, and corresponding deterioration. It is very difficult for a carer to provide care without causing unimaginable pain and immediate, delayed or long term deterioration, unless the light is significantly dimmed.

The more ill I become, the more severe this symptom becomes. As a consequence I have to have very thick, light and sound reducing curtains. Even drawing them causes additional noise pain. The carer, then, has to take into account several different symptoms simultaneously, which is not as easy as it sounds.

My sleep pattern shifts and fluctuates, it is not normal, meaning I need help at odd hours. I can be in a deep asleep at inconvenient moments, making care difficult to provide, you cannot just wake me up as this can cause great harm, shock, deterioration, worsening of symptoms, trigger confusion and disorientation, exacerbate other symptoms.

It is not always possible to tell whether I am asleep or awake and conscious, but in a deep paralysis, unable to communicate this, yet totally aware and needing help.

I frequently have no energy to engage with a carer. I cannot tolerate my limbs being moved by someone else and I cannot move them myself, nor can I tolerate movement, nor being pushed in a wheelchair, so I cannot move from room to room at will, get to the toilet on demand, escape from unpleasant or toxic environments, do what I want, when I want, if at all, get much needed food, get washed, dressed, get help to alleviate physical discomfort from awkward positions, protect myself from noise or light exposure.

Too much energy will be used up in order to just speak even a few words sometimes or make some specific recognisable noise, to indicate that I am conscious, not asleep.

Because of weakness, lack of energy, inability to speak, inability to think or process, paralysis, muscle spasms, breathlessness, difficulty in comprehending questions and finding information or answers in my mind, I often have no ability to communicate specific need. My words and phrases may be limited or come out wrong. The effort can make me sound cross or rude, which does not help.

I have severe to profound levels of cognitive dysfunction that disconnect every simple pathway to communicate and connect with the outside world or another person, This means that I cannot necessarily understand what you say, even if you speak slowly, I may not find the necessary information I need to impart.

If someone speaks too quickly it sounds like a load of gnats biting painfully at my ears, whilst conveying no message or meaning in their content whatsoever; I literally cannot understand it.

Yet I am a sensitive, intelligent person. It must be hard to comprehend how words lose meaning and disappear into nothing in my mind or become an assault.

Communication becomes at best a one way dialogue where I can say some things sometimes, but this varies unpredictably.

Mostly I cannot move. I cannot necessarily tolerate the physical assistance that I am desperate for, whether that is help to eat, to move position, to sit up, to transfer to a wheelchair, to walk with assistance, to get to a toilet.

When paralysed or weakened, I cannot suck from a straw or be sat up to be given a drink despite being desperately thirsty.

I cannot always open my mouth, chew or swallow effectively or at all, even if hungry and this needs understanding, in order to receive help to eat my food, at the right moment.

When I am paralysed, I simply cannot tolerate any sound or movement in the room, let alone physical contact and any attempt to move me will cause physical harm to my muscles and literally torture me.

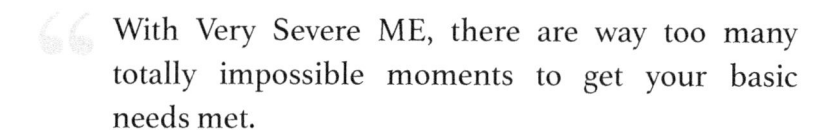

> With Very Severe ME, there are way too many totally impossible moments to get your basic needs met.

2 The only response that helps us, is a MOMENT by MOMENT RESPONSE, in partnership with the person. Any intervention needs to be carefully and tenderly timed, in agreement with me, flowing with me, in order to specifically help me, not make things worse to the point of deterioration that is worse than the extreme situation I am already in.

This requires great flexibility, a willingness to come back at another moment or wait patiently, silently, hopefully with great understanding of the tortured experience I am stuck in. It takes great empathy and compassion to try and comprehend what is being experienced, the issues, the symptoms, the difficulties of engagement and the problems, the pain, plus the devastating consequences that you will cause if you get it wrong.

It takes a gentle and subtle approach. It requires great self-awareness because however quiet and gentle you are, your presence is still going to hurt me. Your actions need to be perfectly timed, for the very best moment that I can bear your help.

Only I know what I can cope with and when I can try and get my need met. Even so, it may still hurt me, because I am never pain-free, but that is my choice to make not yours.

> This is the difference between you seeing me as an object, focusing purely on the task in hand and needing to get it done or seeing me as a person in great need and requiring the right moment to connect with me and flow together as best as possible for me to tolerate the task and get my need met safely in the best way.

I cannot convey how much the slightest wrong thing can cause unimaginable suffering and unnecessary endurance of intolerable levels of pain and other symptom deterioration, due to my profound levels of sensitivity to sound, light, movement, motion, perfume/chemical sensitivity.

The slightest wrong movement, sudden exposure to perfume, light, coughing, talking, clicking, banging or drilling sound, can trigger hours to days of unbearable paralysis, weakened muscles, shaking muscle spasms, intensified pain, massive headache, a completely blank mind, with every thought lost, just like that.

What is worse is knowing that a little extra awareness or care might make the difference between hours of paralysis or not: it is the unnecessary impact of small things that causes great dismay.

> The worst of the most severe end of Severe/ Very Severe ME, where nothing is possible and everything is a torment or a torture, makes accessing much needed care and conveying your needs, with so many broken communication pathways, a massive challenge.

A huge commitment is required to learn and grow consciously together to meet need in the best possible way, accepting that each moment is not equal to the next in terms of tolerability, accessibility, need and possibility.

In the face of such suffering and need, your posture needs to be one of the greatest respect and care.

Remember that this person, before you, in horrendous suffering, extremely ill, with multi-system dysfunction and symptoms affecting every level in their body, is doing their best to bear the unbearable.

They are just like you are on the inside, but with dashed dreams, hopes and complex physical needs, invisible to most people and the world at large.

I have learned that the only way to approach helping me, due to my very severe hypersensitivities, my frequent paralysis, my continuing muscle weakness and profound exhaustion, my inability to tolerate physical contact or sudden movement, surprise or shock, is to very much focus on the MOMENT and to be aware how much pain and torment you can cause me in every moment, if you get it wrong.

All moments, I am in intolerable pain and weakness, with severe to profound hypersensitivities, in a continuum with periodic muscle paralysis and with a mind that is either partially or totally blank, some moments, the presence of another person may be slightly more tolerable, less difficult to bear. Some times I can communicate verbally. Others, it is completely impossible, for the range of reasons given above.

It is in these moments that we have to try and work together, to help me get my needs met. Patience is desperately required on both sides.

We have to accept that there are times that I will have to wait to find the right moment or things will get even worse. The simplest thing, from an external viewpoint, is not simple from within Severe or Very Severe ME. This absolutely has to be remembered. The person with ME must feel in control of what happens to them.

We have found that the right MOMENT brings HELP and alleviates the isolation imposed by the nature of the disease. It is impossible to make demands upon me or for me to comply with external demand or expectation. It simply does not work to take that sort of approach.

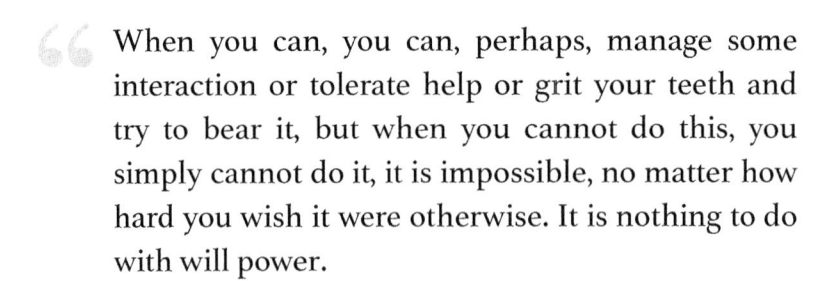

> When you can, you can, perhaps, manage some interaction or tolerate help or grit your teeth and try to bear it, but when you cannot do this, you simply cannot do it, it is impossible, no matter how hard you wish it were otherwise. It is nothing to do with will power.

The problem is that it is not always possible to tell when you can or when you cannot, both from a personal perspective and from the carers view.

There may be times when you might manage but the cost would be too great to tolerate and the after impact devastating or you may feel that you could manage something, you are not sure and yet you might manage it successfully. There will also be times when you absolutely cannot.

Only you can tell this though. This is not something that someone else can judge or encourage you to try harder with.

For people who suffer intensely daily and nightly in this way, I can think of no better or more suitable approach.

All can benefit from their needs being appropriately and gently met at the right and best MOMENT, in a way that honours their illness severity.

If you try to impose care at the wrong moment in the wrong way, without awareness of the hypersensitivities and issues facing the individual with Severe/Very Severe ME, catastrophe will most likely happen and deterioration which can be permanent, may follow.

---

1. Please see Russell Fleming's article : https://meassociation.org.uk/2017/08/severe-me-day-a-time-to-reflect-and-to-consider-what-we-want-to-change-08-august-2017/
2. Never underestimate the difficulties and dangers that a new environment will present to a person with Severe ME. A very gentle, truly person-cantered approach is essential in working a partnership with people who are diagnosed with Severe/Very Severe ME.

    Great harm can be done to the person if their care needs are not carefully considered and respected.

12

MY INVISIBLE WORLD

∼

When you are as ill as you are and as severely disabled with Very Severe ME[1] as you are, even the use of normal aids and equipment that might help other people with disabilities becomes painful or impossible.

The usual assessment processes to get needs met become harder to go through, impossible to navigate or tolerate.

People with Severe/Very Severe ME may be housebound, may also be bed-bound or may be unable to even tolerate being in bed.

> The level of suffering is under-described and unimagined.

The term 'bed-bound', as a measure of severity, without qualifying why, is one that we do not like or agree with; it is behavioural in description, it does not recognise the differences in symptom experience or symptom severity, nor help identify the reasons why the person is in bed.

Unfortunately, it can be used to imply or at least encourage a fatigue focus and description. It is far more helpful, we believe, to recognise the individual symptoms which lead to disability.

They may be individually profound, yet vary significantly in impact between people. Many symptoms are ignored, denied or down-played. As a consequence, people are not provided with the recognition, advice or support they need, to help deal with them.

A Biopsychosocial attitude is irrelevant here; it undermines the physical suffering, the urgent need for physiological explanation, medical respect and a biomedical response.

For example, Noise Sensitivity may be totally disabling, requiring isolation from normality in order to cope. The person may not be in bed, but is still severely disabled and isolated.

It dishonours people's experience, if generalised labels of 'bed-bound' or not, are ascribed as the only measure of severity of illness. Those with profound symptom experience are completely overlooked by this simplistic behavioural terminology.

> Some people may not be bed-bound yet may still be amongst the most severely disabled and struggle/be unable to use even basic aids and equipment.

BELOW ARE some useful descriptions of why a person might be severely disabled with Severe ME and particularly Very Severe ME and how that affects accessing help or even using basic disability aids. It is not necessarily a comprehensive list, just a few examples of what so often is omitted or unidentified and not necessarily understood by others or misinterpreted.

Difficulties posed by ordinary 'taken-for-granted' things, including the use of disability aids, for those most ill and disabled.

WHY DO SOME PEOPLE NEED/HAVE TO STAY IN BED?

- Orthostatic intolerance/dysautonomia
- Blood Pressure issues
- Muscle weakness
- Extreme body and head pain
- Paralysis
- Shaking spasms/tremor
- No energy
- Muscle fatigue
- Difficulty waking up and staying awake
- Need for continued sleep
- Difficulty feeling rested
- Autonomic nervous system dysfunction
- Altered Circadian rhythm cycle, delaying onset of sleep
- A need to rest
- Unrefreshing sleep
- Profound exhaustion
- Nausea/vomiting
- Feeling extremely ill
- Post-exertional deterioration

- Dizziness
- Breathlessness
- Low oxygen
- Difficulty processing environment
- Heart rate variability - Bradychardia and Tachycardia
- Loose joints
- Inability to sit up/be upright

WHY DO SOME PEOPLE NEED TO STAY IN ONE ROOM?

- Safety
- Security
- Need a perfume-free/chemical free environment
- Noise protection to limit exposure
- Light sensitivity requires darkened space
- Comfortably arranged to meet need
- Level of pain incapacitating
- Muscle weakness/stiffness/muscle fatiguability
- Temperature change intolerant
- Decorated minimally to avoid over-stimulation
- No energy to move
- No energy to move about
- Not able to tolerate interaction with others
- Not able to tolerate motion
- Not able to walk any distance or at all
- Not able to physically tolerate sitting or lying in a wheelchair, even if needed
- Intolerant to motion in a wheelchair
- No energy to get dressed

- Unable to use aids and equipment, such as walking sticks, walking frames, for supported movement
- Severe post-exertional deterioration
- Need a noise-reducing environment
- Need a simply decorated, uncluttered environment to avoid over-stimulation
- Closest position to bathroom/toilet
- Cannot move
- Everything is organised to be at hand
- No energy to leave the room
- No ability to be upright or lie down in some cases
- Best/only comfortable seating arrangements in home
- Stuck upstairs unable to get down
- Needs can only be met in a limited space
- Controlled environment
- Not generally able to be with other people in the home or tolerate background noise or interaction
- Outdoor environment may be too bright, too noisy, too chemically/perfume contaminated, too overwhelming cognitively or visually or unsafe surfaces, steps, bumps, unsound ground etc

DIFFICULTIES WITH STAIR LIFTS

- Expensive, may be unfordable
- Stairs may be too steep or an awkward shape to have one installed
- Noise of a motor may be too much to tolerate for people with severe noise sensitivity
- Motion may be intolerable

- May be unsafe due to muscle weakness to sit up or endure movement safely
- Possible smell of oil for people with MCS endangers health
- May not have a strong enough handgrip ability due to muscle weakness/pain in hands
- May be paralysed and unable to bear any contact or movement
- Pain may be too severe to tolerate motion or movement
- Seat may not offer enough back support or leg support
- May not be strong enough to operate it independently
- Dizziness may make it unbearable
- Nausea may make motion intolerable
- May not be able to safely transfer onto seat and off again
- Cognitive dysfunction may make it hard to use or remember how to use
- Too ill to deal with people for services and breakdowns etc

DIFFICULTY WITH SHOWERING

- Difficulty getting out of bed or off seat to get to bathroom/shower room.
- Difficulty getting to the bathroom/shower room due to muscle weakness, muscle fatigue, post- exertional neuro-immune reaction, paralysis, co-ordination difficulties

- Not enough energy to undress, let alone get in a shower and wash
- Difficulty transferring to a shower chair or bath-board over a bath
- Difficulty with hardness of shower chair seat or bath-board causing pain or exacerbating existing levels of pain
- Difficulty getting in and out of shower for a variety of different symptom experiences
- Unable to turn shower on or off
- Difficulty maintaining water heat at tolerable level.
- Risk of burning with hot water or getting too cold with cold water variability
- A shower over a bath may cause more access problems than a walk-in shower
- Inability to stand or safely sit, unsteady on feet even with support
- Not enough energy to endure the whole process of getting in and out of shower and washing and drying oneself, even with help.
- Extreme pain may make physical contact of falling water on skin an unbearable agony
- Shock of water on skin may act as a shock to intensify symptoms
- Head-pain may not tolerate contact of water
- Getting too cold once shower stops
- Hypersethesia making contact from water unbearable or drying with a towel too painful
- Needing a dark room may make the environment not safe to shower in
- Noise of water falling may be intolerable if sound sensitive

- Noise of motor may be too loud and cause pain, headache, upset, intolerance, paralysis, muscle shaking or other symptom deterioration
- Noise from an extractor fan may be too loud to tolerate

DIFFICULTY WITH DECORATING

- Unable to do it yourself
- Noise
- Chemical exposure
- Perfume exposure
- Inability to tolerate people in the house or room
- Difficulty of people wearing perfumed products contaminating environment further
- Lack of energy or cognitive ability to arrange and cope with the process
- Poverty: low odour paints can be extremely expensive
- Inability to leave the room or the house that needs decorating in order for it to proceed
- The length of time required to do the work may take too long even if someone can cope with the extra issues for a little time
- Unpredictability and unreliability of people helping, coming on time and sticking to agreed times
- Finding helpers who understand your illness and who are willing to be flexible
- Impossibility of cleaning up afterwards or coping with upheaval and changes to routine
- Post-exertional deterioration
- Risk of new symptoms developing

DIFFICULTY WITH GETTING NEW THINGS

- Inability to go to a shop to try something out to check if it is comfortable or suits your need
- Unpredictability of online buying, measuring, colour accuracy, inability to tell comfortability, texture of material, chemical or perfume smell of product or wrapping
- Lack of physical ability or energy to open packaging or send things back if unsuitable
- Inability to deal with sales person online or on telephone or in person, due to severity of illness, headache, head pain, communication difficulties, no energy to speak or comprehend, noise sensitivity, cognitive difficulties, inability to speak or find words and phrases needed, too slow to process conversation or articulate issues
- Too ill to deal with delivery of product, especially if you live alone and are bed-bound or stuck on a chair unable to get off it
- Cannot tolerate the door bell ringing
- Cannot sign for goods
- Cannot tell what time a parcel will be delivered to ensure someone is there to avoid noise, light, chemical, perfume exposure or other extra stresses that deteriorate symptoms
- Difficulty unpacking purchase if weak hands, no strength, no ability to move it or try it on or put it where it needs to go
- Vulnerability of chemical smells from new products

which take many months to wear off and can endanger health
- Difficulty tolerating other people's presence in the room or house even if you have someone willing and able to help you
- Not enough energy to explain your need to someone else in order for them to help you in the right way
- Someone else cannot tell how a product feels or whether the texture, smells, whether the colour/brightness of colour is okay for your eyes to tolerate, whether it has a noise, if mechanical - you need to do it yourself, but cannot
- Not knowing whether it will inadvertently trigger an allergic reaction

DIFFICULTY WITH USING A WHEELCHAIR

- Not everyone will be able to sit upright or lean back at an angle in a wheelchair for different reasons: eg orthostatic intolerance/dysautonomia, muscle weakness or stiffness, extreme pain, loose joints, muscle spasms and tremor, periodic or permanent paralysis, dizziness
- Some may need to lie completely flat or have appropriate padding to get comfortable at the right angle; everyone will not be the same or use may be variably possible
- Some may not tolerate using a wheelchair even with very limited mobility, due to the nature and severity of symptoms and impact of motion
- Motion, both forward and/or backward, may be intolerable to some

- Being tipped backwards may be unbearable, especially with dysautonomia
- A jolt to the chair or a bump may be excruciating, deteriorative, unbearable, trigger shock or paralysis, increase pain, cause irritation, confusion or upset
- It may be hard to get a seat that is soft enough or padded enough in the right places or with surfaces that are bearable with contact
- New smells or chemicals and cushioning materials may be an issue for people with MCS
- Cushions must be supportive yet soft enough for comfort and may not be possible to find anything suitable if extremely pressure sensitive, hypersensitive or in severe pain.
- Texture of fabric may also be an important barrier or chemicals and dyes
- Professionals may not understand the importance or need to use a wheelchair, especially if it is not always required or variably tolerated or possible to use and the post-exertional impact of having or not having one or the potential for long term deterioration, is not visible until it is too late
- It is not easy to get a design that suits someone with severe pressure sensitivity, high pain or hyperesthesia or postural issues
- It is hard to get a wheelchair that does not have hard front wheels, but rather has pneumatic tyres to minimise bumps
- Electric chairs may be impossible to control independently due to muscle weakness, lack of co-ordination or poor co-ordination, poor vision, post-exertional deterioration, lack of energy, muscle or

nerve pain, lack of stamina, poor spatial awareness, cognitive issues like slow processing of environmental information
- There may be difficulty physically charging or safely charging batteries for electric wheelchairs if there is limited space
- Ramps, path width outdoors or corridor/room space indoors and access are often issues to be considered
- Wheelchair maintenance can be extremely difficult and it may not be possible to cope with someone else doing it for you

DIFFICULTY ENGAGING WITH PEOPLE IN ORDER TO GET NEEDS MET

- People may be too ill to speak or move or convey their need even
- People may be too noise sensitive to tolerate another persons voice, both loudness and tone, their laughter or even a whisper, the sounds they make when moving their body, whilst making gestures or their footsteps in the room or on the stairs or the banging of doors, even if quietly shut or opened, may be too much to tolerate and risk deterioration
- People may not know how to safely and effectively communicate especially if sign language or silence and waiting is required
- A door bell can be incapacitating, painful, harmful, deteriorative to someone with severe sound sensitivity and the inability to answer or stop the sound can be disturbing, painful or exacerbating
- People may be too weak and limited in energy to

move, think, talk, debate, answer questions, ask questions, find words, understand information, sit up, stand, explain, open windows to air rooms if perfume-exposed, unable to open curtains to let in light if needed, due to physical inability as well photophobia
- Chemical and perfume sensitivity and allergy are real barriers to being with people or allowing them into the room or the home
- Some people may be physically paralysed or near to paralysis, unable to communicate or tolerate anyone's presence, may appear asleep, when actually conscious and awake, yet unable to move or open their eyes.
- Clothing rustling, with another person's movement, can be a torment to a person with severe/profound noise sensitivity
- People who gesticulate or move quickly about may cause pain, confusion, deterioration due to movement sensitivity
- People with Severe ME may sometimes suddenly, unpredictably and unexpectedly completely run out of energy, deteriorate, develop severe pain, headache, blank mind, nausea, vomiting, paralysis or other symptom increase and no longer be able to engage in conversation or bear company in the room, may only have very limited time before this happens, if engagement is possible at all and will have strict regimes and specific needs, to cope in these circumstances, but not necessarily be able to convey them
- A person with Severe ME may not be able to follow

conversation especially if there is any background noise
- It may not be possible to tolerate more than one person at a time in the room
- Using phones or keyboards/ computers/ tablets, may be variable to impossible to use for communication purposes, depending on the ability to tolerate magnets, holding the implement, reading, typing, sound, speaking a message, even with the possible use of particular aids to help, such as voice activation programs, as these still may not be practicable to use, as they may take too much cognitive or physical effort. There may be problems with co-ordination, holding things or fine movement, making staying in touch with others or communicating vital needs very difficult indeed, especially if one to one time is not tolerable or possible or severely limited
- Someone putting the slightest pressure, not just on the person, but on the bed or wheelchair or seat, leaning on it, for example, can literally cause pain and weakening and should never be done without agreement, if at all, yet how easily this can be done by an unaware visitor, without any understanding of the dire impact
- If speech is tolerated, it may need to be extremely slow, with no complex phrases, may need to use simple language, quietly spoken, may need long pauses between sentences to enable processing to occur, may for some, need to be repeated, especially if spoken too fast the first time or it may be that only once is the limit, so comprehension is lost and

conversation halted, especially if there are a lot of words to deal with
- Questions may be impossible to answer for a variety of different reasons, such as difficulty comprehending the question, difficulty finding information to reply, difficulty articulating the response, even if the information has been found. The effort of even thinking about the answer may cause further shutting down of the minds ability to think or retrieve information or communicate and may make physical symptoms worse or trigger symptoms unexpectedly, such as muscle spasms, severe headache etc
- Visualisation or following description or information from someone else, may not be possible, making it hard to follow conversation and have two-way interaction
- There is a post-exertional reaction not only to physical exertion but also to cognitive effort, which can result in an even blanker mind than the norm, for the person, making communication even more difficult to achieve and potentially jeopardising the possibility of essential communication in the near and/or long term future
- Physical contact, even light contact, whether expected or unexpected, may cause shock, intense pain, paralysis, shaking muscle spasms, exacerbation of other symptoms and could be unintentionally catastrophic to the person affected in this way
- The sudden exposure to noise, such as a sudden mobile phone ring or an object accidentally knocked

over or dropped, a sneeze, a cough, even a head scratch, can negatively impact some, which brings an extra problem in interacting with anyone
- There is an extra vulnerability to catching viruses from visitors, which brings an added risk and a particular additional issue to be aware of, in order to safe-guard health from worsening and may not always be fully thought through or the high risk to health completely understood by others
- A person in the room may not understand the specific and complex needs of the person and how their direct presence can create extra difficulties or deterioration from the subtlest thing, nor how to respond; they may not realise or recognise their cognitive impact, for example, that can limit language, memory, information understanding, nor comprehend the harm that ensues if the person's reality is ignored or not understood, is not known or accepted
- People with Severe ME are likely to have multiple breaks to communication and may struggle to engage with people at all. They require an extremely aware, sensitive approach and an acute understanding of their genuine difficulties in getting even their most basic needs met.

---

1. With Severe /Very Severe ME, typically you find are on your own; finding some way to survive the never-ending onslaught of multiple physical symptoms, moment by outlandish moment, is beyond impossible.

    You might be lucky and have an aware GP - but they are unlikely to have access to expert help, so the GP is very limited in how they can help.

    You might be able to pay privately, but that is fraught with risk.

    This is the stark situation people with Severe /Very Severe ME are in.

13

AN INTRODUCTION TO SEVERE ME: A CONUNDRUM OF CARE

This very powerful article was published by the ME Association [1] in 2020 and has been reproduced with kind permission of the Author, who we have known for many years despite having never met physically due to the severity of illness

---

1. The ME Association https://meassociation.org.uk/

14

SEVERE ME A CONUNDRUM IN CARE BY EIRA STUART

∼

S EVERE M.E. POSES A definitive conundrum to residential care providers. It may seem on first impression that the patient's needs are too complex, particularly in the very severe cases. It is entirely possible to accommodate however, M.E. care does not and cannot adhere to standard procedures in care.

As such, a fundamental understanding of the illness is firstly needed and appropriate and necessary adjustments to the patients needs must be provided. M.E. sufferers need stability and continuity in care, this is dedicated individualised care which should only be carried out by compassionate experienced carers.

My recommendation to those considering residential care would be to try to remain at home as far as possible and obtain as much community support as possible. An M.E. patient is likely to have more control over their environment in their own home and be subject to less policies and procedures in a domestic setting. This advice is likely to serve some patients better than others due to the variability in quality and level of care that is available in each region.

There are currently no specialist support services for M.E. patients. Hospitals are potential disaster zones which could make M.E. patients worse due to the lack of necessary adaptions, the highly stimulating atmosphere and general ignorance of medical professionals.

In response to my query regarding suitable residential care for M.E. patients, the M.E. Association affirms that:

"Specialist nursing care with quiet-running and chemical-free facilities would need to be provided for people with moderate to severe M.E. I regret to have to tell you that there are no such places known to us in the U.K.

There have been two attempts by charities to set up respite care and longer-term homes for people with M.E. in the last twenty years and both failed. In each case, the charities concerned were unable to persuade either the NHS or an existing social care provider to come into the project as a partner. There were also huge annual running costs attached to each scheme which the charities could not sustain on their own."

Consequently, M.E. patients struggle to receive care funding, let alone residential funding, or NHS Continuing Health Care funding. The situation is unlikely to be resolved until the biomedical realty of M.E. is nationally recognised among clinicians and the appropriate funding apportioned for specialist care.

Severe M.E. sufferer Dr Andrew McLellan, is a former biologist who was recently interviewed for a podcast on living well with chronic illness *This is Not What I Ordered* hosted by

Lauren Selfridge. He shared his views with me on the current challenges faced by M.E. patients in care:

"It is not just people with severe M.E. who get confined to homes for the elderly once we go beyond community care. The charity Sue Ryder estimates that around 15 000 people in the UK are in this situation due to the lack of facilities for younger adults with severe chronic conditions*.

Something clearly needs to be done. Education is the most obvious, but also regional homes for adults who need care due to ongoing disability and illness."

Prior to admission to a nursing home, it would be worth spending some time getting to know the place. I would not recommend going on blind faith or on the basis of verbal agreements which are not legally binding. I would recommend speaking to the nurses and senior carer(s). Be aware that managers may not be active on the floor during shifts and will have less of an idea of how the shift is run than the actual people on the ground: the carers. Find out who is in charge of allocations, is it the nurse or the senior carers? How involved are the nurses?

Do they have an active role in care, or do they only see patients to give medications and carry out invasive nursing tasks? If so, the patient could end up never seeing a nurse which means they will be primarily cared for by the carers. Ask how allocations are done. What sort of shift patterns does the home adopt? How often are carers rotated between wings and between floors and most importantly carer to patient ratios. It may also be worth asking what strategies are in place in circumstances of short staffing.

Short staffing is a problem that pervades the care industry. It goes with the territory to have a moderately high turn over rate of staff. Sadly, care is treated as an industry rather than a vocation. This is an issue that needs to be seriously addressed by the health minister and by local councils and MPs. More and more complex conditions are being managed in the community or in nursing homes rather than in hospitals. So it is necessary for care to be properly regulated and established as a skilled vocation with minimum standards of skill (ideally NVQ3 for nursing home staff and NVQ 2 for social carers) literacy (Atleast 6 GCSEs and 2-3 A levels or a Dip HE or higher) and commensurate wages if national care standards are to be improved.

It is necessary for all M.E. patients to be aware that the average person has never heard of M.E. or only has a vague idea and usually only of the milder cases who are able to self care, even work. Severe M.E. is an entirely different kettle of fish and only 25% of M.E. patients are severely affected.

It is therefore imperative to ascertain how willing a prospective provider is to train a small group of carers or to provide continuity in care. What kind of training do they give staff? Are they willing to accommodate M.E. specific training on an on going basis for example: bi-annually? Ensure all agreements are put in writing prior to admission. Find out the nurses attitudes to M.E. Do they adopt the mistaken biopsychosocial (BPS) approach? Are they willing to take direction from an M.E. specialist consultant?

It would be ideal if staff from the home could attend the M.E. patients home and observe their care. In addition to this, I would also recommend writing a care plan in advance of admission, including a shorter care summary document in bullet points outlining the patients routine.

Nursing homes as institutions are bound by certain principles of "good practice" in various areas including manual handling, health and safety and infection control, to name but a few. They have certain guidelines they must adhere to which are mandated by Care Quality Commission (CQC), the care regulator in the U.K.

Nursing homes are obliged to vacuum on a daily basis for infection control, mattresses are expected to be turned every week. They also have a duty to safeguard the welfare of staff, therefore beds will need to be set a at a safe height for manual handling. It is important to consider what kind of bed the patient would need. Are they able to be hoisted to have the mattress turned regularly? Are vibrations from electric beds likely to exacerbate symptoms?

If so, indemnity will need to be put in place so that the home is not penalised by the CQC for failing to adhere to standard protocol. The patient will also require a bed with low maintenance that can be kept at one height.

There are currently no stipulations in Health and Safety laws as to the minimum requirement of light. The Disability Law Service advises that if light is "injurious to health", then the institution has a disability equality duty to make reasonable adjustments in line with the Disability Equality Act. However, they also have a duty to maintain a safe working environment for staff, so a balance between both factors will need to be found. If the M.E. patient is severely light sensitive, this is a parameter that must be gaged in advance to avoid problems upon admission. Both the nursing home and the patients should consider the following:

Is the patient sensitive to light? If so to what extent? Do they require a blacked out room, are they likely to be affected by light coming in from under the door in the hallway? Will they need to have this light off? Is the home, able to accommodate this or must lights remain on continuously for health and safety purposes including at night? Can they be switched off at night?

If not could a fireproof curtain be installed to mitigate this? This would also circumvent the increase of light when carers enter the room.

If the patient is particularly light or noise sensitive then it is advisable to house them in a room at the end of the corridor or in quiet low traffic areas away from noisy communal areas such as dining rooms/lounges/kitchen or laundry facilities. Draughts from hallway windows should also be considered if the patient has problems with thermoregulation. Shower rooms need to be kept ventilated and any in the vicinity are likely to cause a draught.

If the room overlooks a car park is the coming and going of cars likely to impact the patient?

If the room overlooks the garden you may need to discuss whether the lawn mower will affect the patient. Considerations would also need to be made regarding the neighbouring residents. Are they loud do they shout or call out? Would the home be able to install sound panels to sound proof the rooms? Do neighbouring residents have air mats with pumps likely to make noise? Is there any noise from pipes above below or in the walls.

It is standard practice in nursing homes for residents to be washed daily, bathed weekly and to receive several pad changes a day. This level of care could be counterproductive, even harmful to a severe M.E. patient who may only be able to be washed in bed once a week or even only once a month. Hoisting and removing such a patient to bathe could be fatal for a severely affected patient who may be severely movement intolerant and only able to tolerate minimum care. Jodi Basset founder of the Hummingbird Foundation for M.E. stated: Increasing cardiac output by even 1% in a severe M.E. could be fatal (Cheney in Bassett 2011:60).

In this case the nursing home will need documentation to indemnify themselves against potential allegations of neglect for not providing the standard level of care given to other residents. A confirmation of mental capacity will ensure the patient is protected from forcible care interventions or deprivation of liberties (DoLs).

An individualised person centred approach therefore factors greatly in M.E. care. A carer cannot merely execute a list of care tasks. They need to have an understanding of how M.E. affects this particular patient. What is their best time of day? What is their baseline activity tolerance? Do they suffer from paresis/paralysis? Is it permanent paralysis in the legs? Transient paresis of the arms? Paralysis that is exacerbated by exertion? Do they have seizures? Do they suffer from Relapsing/Remitting M.E. or Secondary progressive? Are they light sensitive? Noise sensitive? Touch sensitive? Do their arms or legs give out or lose function when moved around? Is one side more functional then the other? Do their tolerance levels change throughout the day?

Some M.E. patients are so ill that they cannot be touched or moved repetitively or multiple times due to muscle fatigability, orthostatic intolerance, Postural orthostatic Tachycardia Syndrome (PoTS) dysautonomia and neurally mediated hypotension. If this is the case, then the home may need to apply extended manual handling procedures and staff will need to be trained in this area.

On the other hand, there are severely affected M.E. patients who require extensive physical care to the point of needing a care visit every two to three hours or more times a day, particularly if they are tube fed. This will of course be impossible for those with severe sensory hypersensitivities and this is in fact where two severe patients can defer despite both being severe.

An M.E. sufferer who is bed bound lives in a prison from which they cannot escape. Their nervous systems are highly sensitive, their fight or flight mechanism is on overdrive, they are weak and vulnerable, they feel as though they have the flu, everything hurts, migraines, seizures, tremors, myoclonus, blindness, paresis, paralysis, both permanent and transient, myasthenia gravis like symptoms, muscle fatigability, their skin and body may burn throb or pulse, dysautonomia makes them feel sea sick and as though they are moving and rocking even when totally motionless, ringing in the ears, sensory overload, sensory storms, brain fog, difficulty concentrating, memory lapses, disorientation, most of these constant and unrelenting, others activity induced. It is a lot to live with all the time:

"how can I convey to you that I live in a totally different world than you, even if I'm in the same room as you, even if you appear to be in the same physical space as me, believe me I am not experiencing anything in the same way as you" (Crowhurst 2018:33).... *"it is more than torment, more than torture, more than indescribable, more than intolerable, more than unacceptable, more than completely unbearable. It is screamingly hostile and negating. It is barbaric in its cruelty. It is exquisitely diminishing. It is almost completely incomprehensible in its agony it is so vast, so punishing, so pure, so bleak, so full of sensations that are beyond endurance."* (Crowhurst 2018:26).

∼

REFERENCES:

-*This is not what I ordered* (2019) December [podcast]. Available at: https://ayearinzen.home.blog/podcast-interview/?

fbclid=IwAR2zeqWi2mDXwbJ12NP1dQJgdTK3mHH2-P6WSQlPEx1BUb1utZUVbL3JijA

-Burns, R. And Simmons, E. (2019) *She's a high-achieving teacher who defied multiple sclerosis to travel all over the world. So why HAS Nina been left to rot in an old people's home at just 46?*. The Mail on Sunday, 20 August. Available at: https://www.dailymail.co.uk/health/article-7317591/Why-multiple-sclerosis-sufferer-Nina-left-rot-old-peoples-home-just-46.html-Bassett,J., *Caring for the Severe M.E. Patient.* Lulu: 2011.

Crowhurst G., *Caring For ME, a pocketbook course for carers.* Lulu: 2018.

-Stuart, E., Severe *M.E. Day: Life in a Nursing Home, Light Sensitivity and Very Severe M.E.* The M.E. Association, August 2019:

https://www.meassociation.org.uk/2019/08/severe-me-day-life-in-a-nursing-home-light-sensitivity-and-very-severe-m-e-by-eira-stuart-08-august-2019/

INTRODUCTION TO THE MONSTROUS STING IN THE TAIL

As their website says, the Hope 4 ME & Fibro Charity[1] began many years ago, as a thought by Treasurer and Founder Joan McParland.

Today Hope 4 ME & Fibro Northern Ireland regularly hosts ground breaking patient and medical conferences that bring international expertise to Northern Ireland, raises funding for Bio-Medical research, liaises with all major ME and Fibromyalgia charities, both in UK and Ireland and constantly seeks to raise awareness.

It is a huge honour for me to include this contribution by Joan, for whom I have immense respect. It is not always easy to articulate and write about Severe ME, especially when in a 'bad crash', as Joan was when she wrote this. It takes massive effort and patience.

Writing a few lines every day, until it was complete, Joan's piece contrasts the underfunded, under-researched response to the invisible, neglected, stigmatised disease, ME, where you are left to "sink or swim alone", in comparison to the response to Covid 19.

---

1. Joan McParland's vision is to establish specialist NHS services in Northern Ireland for all ME and Fibromyalgia patients . Please see the Hope4ME & Fibro Charity website: https://hope4mefibro.org/about/

16

THE MONSTROUS STING IN THE TAIL OF MYALGIC ENCEPHALOMYELITIS BY JOAN MCPARLAND

∼

MY THOUGHTS ON HOW it's hard to decide which actual sting in the tail of M.E. is the worst.......

Is it the fact there's no cure?

No, this is the case in most if not all chronic diseases.

Is it the fact there's no effective treatment?

No, this is the case in most chronic diseases.

Is it the fact there's no definitive diagnostic test?

No, because some other diseases too, need expert clinical judgement alongside testing to reach secure diagnoses.

Is it the fact, sometimes you will outwardly appear well?

No, many diseases are invisible.

Is it the fact, except for your family, no one will witness the extent of your suffering?

No, many patients with chronic illnesses are bed/house bound and cut off from the outside world.

Is it the fact that our lives are turned upside down and losses occur in every aspect of previous healthy living i.e. loss of careers, financial security, family life, social life, independence and the ability of personal self care?

No, this happens in varying degrees with many chronic diseases.

The sting:

Is it that no other disease is so grossly underfunded by governments and M.E. patients have no other choice than to find the money themselves, to invest in whichever biomedical research facilities, look like giving us the best chance in finding answers?

Yes.

Is it the disbelief and dismissal when we turn to healthcare providers for help?

Yes.

Is it the mental torture of being told you're just making it up, as the disease doesn't even exist?

Yes.

Is it the long-standing stigma we can't seem to overcome no matter how hard we try to educate others, including members of the healthcare profession?

Yes.

Is it the fact WHO classified M.E. is still not included during medical training?

Yes.

Is it because your determination and efforts to take part in life, make you more ill?

Yes.

Is it because, when not completely bed-bound, you will get times when the illness dupes you into thinking you are well enough to escape.... and have that coffee or meal out with family or friends or grocery shop or go to the cinema or hairdressers or whatever makes your heart sing? You may well achieve these goals sometimes but all times, either immediately you do escape or a day or two later, you will pay dearly.

Yes.

Is it the memory of the day, unable to hold your head up to answer the questions being fired, by five sickness benefit assessors, as they sat round your bed and you wept after two hours of interrogation, when an independent observer told your husband to "let her answer herself," as he watched your depleting energy and distress and tried to help?

Yes.

Is it the day a year ago, when a medical professional said he KNEW you'd just needed GET/CBT all along?

Yes.

Is it the fact that you use every molecule of physical energy and cognitive ability to overcome all of these things above, yet they seem always so close, yet so far away from any meaningful breakthroughs?

Yes.

Or is it now, during a pandemic with half of the planet trapped in their homes, all of the life saving things you'd asked for, for 20 years, are available without any 'fight.'?

Free online courses to help with mental health during isolation, loneliness, ill-health.

Governments investing in suicide prevention schemes for traumatised nations and research into post-Covid 'fatigue.'

Energy saving telephone consultations with doctors, organisations ensuring food essentials are delivered to your door and random acts of kindness from strangers.

Yet, the stigma of M.E. and the rest, prevented these things we'd needed for decades and we were left to sink or swim alone.

I'm glad for all who made it.

INTRODUCTION TO ACCESSIBILITY AND CREATIVITY: A REVIEW OF INTO THE LIGHT, ARTIST BOOK IN A BOX BY CORINA DUYN

THE FOLLOWING IS WRITTEN in loving thanks for Corina Duyn's kindness and friendship. A deep sense of connection is so important to find, both for the person with Severe ME, who is cut off from most normal, ordinary things and Carers, who have to immerse their own lives too in the isolation and separation from society.

It is very important to remember that despite severe, even profound symptom experience, people with Severe and Very Severe ME may also have a wonderful range of talents and a deep need to find connection and recognition.

They are so much more than their illness, even when that illness is devastating, intense, often overwhelming and incurable, with multiple physical and cognitive dysfunctions and broken communication pathways.

18

ACCESSIBILITY AND CREATIVITY A REVIEW OF INTO THE LIGHT, ARTISTS BOOK IN A BOX BY CORINA DUYN

> 'Her pain is terrible today, her tears a fire, it is impossible to see the soft summer
> morning's beauty, the gentle shadows, such is her agony.
> Another day lost.
> I have run out of words to pray.'

~

On a day when my devoted husband wrote these pain-filled words and the day indeed seemed impossible to bear and utterly lost, a wonderful gift popped through the letterbox on to our mat, the timing of which was perfect.

To back track a little, whilst looking for inspiration for Severe ME Understanding and Remembrance Day 2017, we unexpectedly and I have to say, to my surprise and delight, discovered a previously unseen piece of writing on a Disability

Arts Online web page, that included a mention of my name and my Stick Picture art.

Thrilled

I confess that having been thrown into worsening unimaginable levels of repeated paralysis, for the last 7 years, my mind had forgotten, unbelievably, even that I had drawn them. *I was in fact, it has to be said, thrilled to be mentioned and recognised as an artist by another artist. It reawakened a light in me and was such a wonderful affirmation.*

Excitingly, it led us to the beautiful, tender, gentle world and imagery of Corina Duyn, her art, puppetry and writings, were revealed to us through birdsong and nature and a beautifully presented web site: a stunningly innovate, determined and exquisitely detailed artist, with, an extra dimension of knowing, brought about by, to my amazement, her immersion of necessity into the world of Severe ME.

Fourteen years of solitude and being still with nature, in order to cope with her illness, her art, her life, her expression of wisdom through everything she does, struck a chord in my heart. It resonated deep.

It inspired. It uplifted, it sang a song of hope in the depth of my pain-filled, noise racked, hypersensitive body, it reminded me not only of what I knew, echoing back from what she also knew, but also who I was in the core of my being, a free spirit, an artist, someone who ultimately has been trying to climb out of the pit that I have been thrown into and unwantingly captured in, by a desperately serious and very severe form of Myalgic Encephalomyelitis, myself.

Beauty I can appreciate

Reading books has been way beyond me for decades now. Limited coordination, visual disturbance, eye pain, cognitive dysfunction, physical disability and a continuum with paralysis have rendered books beyond me. Yet beauty, I can appreciate, imagery I can feel, colour and nature can touch me. Short phrases and words can at the right time, in the right way, be comprehended.

Stillness is essential. Healing is a path. Hope is elusive, yet necessary, to keep going. Inspiration, kindness, caring, the hope of strangers, the compassion and knowing of one too who has known, the unexpected generosity of a gift tenderly offered, is an incredible lifeline, especially when you live in total isolation from the world and the invisibility of your moment by moment suffering mostly feels overwhelming, 25 years on.

So into our silent world, when our need for beauty was great, came Corina Duyn's incredible ' *Into the Light Artist Book in a Box*'.

Our first impressions of this wonderful book in a box were how incredibly beautiful it looks and what a beautiful presentation and fantastic idea it is!

There is a video about it on Corina's website, however even this does not do full justice to the exquisitely beautiful book that arrived in the post. Corina also has several You Tube videos from which you can gain more insight into her work. For instance, the book was three years in the making and was inspired by the simplicity of Tibetan Prayer flags, fluttering in the breeze.

With ME things are never straight forward. There seems to be a lot of waiting involved, limiting the time possible to proactively create the desired image. Then there is the practicality of how, how to do that which you can see in your mind, how to bring it into the Light! Corina is a total inspiration to me, someone who has experienced many of the things that I too have known.

She has found healing over the years, though not well and in great pain and found a way to express and share her knowledge and wisdom, simply, purely and effectively through art, through writing, through photography and nature, puppets, tapestry, poetry, emerging into the Light from the depth of solitude, brought to her by this path of illness, with birds as her companions and inspiration.

Deconstructed and elegant

The Book in a Box is a uniquely brilliant gift! It is so much more accessible to me and hopefully to others who also struggle with more complex visual difficulties, cognitive dysfunction, muscle weakness and a host of other symptoms that make connection, comprehension and communication so impossibly hard.

Knowing Corina has been so affected by ME for many years and has gained great insight herself, creates a unique bond for others struggling and coping with similar circumstance.

What we love about this in essence deconstructed and elegantly transformed book, is how it brings accessibility, where an ordinary book is too heavy, too complex and often too many pages and too many words to manage. This book, which comes in four different versions, is a box of exquisitely designed single pages that increases accessibility to the words and images within.

Here a single sheet is light to hold, or can sit lightly on the lap when numb empty fingers cannot hold it.

The imagery and photography convey so much to me personally - they elicit a recognition and deep resonance in my heart of my own experience, yet bring hope. They seem to bring a multidimensional aspect because it resonates so deeply with what I know myself also from my own very severe illness and helps me recognises a bond of knowing between us, carried through the messages, words, imagery, beyond what is physically seen - the gift of not aloneness, the comprehension of pain, the need to surrender to the experience yet not to give in, the triumph, the resilience of the human heart and spirit despite intense physical suffering.

We wish Corina every success with this wonderful healing Book in a Box and all her other amazing artwork.

Thank you Corina for the inspiration and love in its pages.

19

INTRODUCTION TO EMILY'S APPEAL.

This poignant appeal for proper research and proper care, for those severely affected by ME, was written in 2011 by the late Emily Collingridge. It is still just as relevant today.

20

AN APPEAL, BY EMILY COLLINGRIDGE

∼

I developed the neurological condition Myalgic Encephalomyelitis (ME) when I was 6 years old. In April 2011 I turned 30. I still have ME.

ME coloured every aspect of my childhood; it painfully restricted my teens and it completely destroyed my twenties. Now, as I move into the next decade of my life, I am more crippled than ever by this horrific disease.

My doctors tell me that I have been pushed to the greatest extremes of suffering that illness can ever push a person. I have come very close to dying on more than one occasion. If you met me you may well think I was about to die now - it's like that every single day. After all these years **I still struggle to understand how it's possible to feel so ill so relentlessly.**

My reaction to small exertions and sensory stimulation is extreme. For example, voices wafting up from downstairs, a brief doctor's visit, a little light, all can leave me with surging pain, on the verge of vomiting, struggling with each breath and feeling I'll go mad with the suffering. Of course it can also be as bad as this for no particular reason - and often is. I cannot be washed, cannot raise my head, cannot have company, cannot be lifted from bed, cannot look out of the window, cannot be touched, cannot watch television or listen to music - the list is long. **ME has made my body an agonising prison.**

My days and nights are filled with restless sleep interspersed with injections, needle changes (for a syringe driver), nappy changes (as well as experiencing transient paralysis and at times being blind and mute, I am doubly incontinent) and medicines/fluid being pumped into my stomach through a tube. My life could be better if I had a Hickman line (line which goes into a major vein and sits in the heart) for IV drugs and fluids, but such a thing would likely kill me. I'm on a huge cocktail of strong medications which help, yet still most days **the suffering is incomprehensible.** During the worst hours I may go without the extra morphine I need as I feel so ill that the thought of my mother coming near to administer it is intolerable - this despite **pain levels so high that I hallucinate.** I live in constant fear of a crisis driving me into hospital; our hospitals have shown such lack of consideration for the special needs of patients like me that time spent in hospital is torture (eased only by the incredible kindness shown by some nurses and doctors) and invariably causes further deterioration.

Many days I feel utter despair.

But, unlike some sufferers, over the years in which I've had severe ME (the illness began mildly and has taken a progressive course) I have at least had periods of respite from the worst of it. During those periods I was still very ill, but it was possible to enjoy something of life. So in these dark days I know there is a real chance of better times ahead and that keeps me going.

My entire future, and the greatly improved health I so long for, however, currently hinges on luck alone. This is wrong. As I lie here, wishing and hoping and simply trying to survive, I (and the thousands like me - this is not a rare illness) should at least have the comfort of knowing that there are many, many well-funded scientists and doctors who are pulling out all the stops in the quest to find a treatment which may restore my health and that the NHS is doing all possible to care for me as I need to be cared for - but I don't. **This wretched, ugly disease is made all the more so through the scandalous lack of research into its most severe form and the lack of necessary, appropriate support for those suffering from it.** This is something that must change.

And that is why I tell my story; why I fight my painfully debilitated body to type this out on a smartphone one difficult sentence at a time and to make my appeal to governments, funders, medical experts and others: **please put an end to the abandonment of people with severe ME and give us all real reason to hope.**

∼

YOU CAN SUPPORT Emily's cause and everyone with severe ME by viewing the "Severe ME/CFS: A Guide to Living" Facebook page at www.facebook.com/severemecfsguide Both sufferers and non sufferers welcome! See also www.severeME.info.

Both provide information on simple ways to help ensure that everyone with severe ME and all the professionals and loved ones involved in their care have access to "Severe ME/CFS: A Guide to Living" which is the most comprehensive source of advice on coping with all aspects of life with severe ME and has been described as "what every sufferer has been waiting for" (by a patient), "literally life changing" (by a carer) and "essential reading for anyone treating a patient with severe ME" (by a professional).

(C) Emily Collingridge 2010-2011

21

IT WOULD NOT BE SO

∽

My life
Is a living torment
I wish it were not so
I wish I could say
That everything I had tried to do to get well had
 helped me
But it would not be so
I wish I could say
That every one who tried to help me had done so
But it would not be so
I wish I could say that everyone I trusted had been
 worthy of it
But it would not be so
I wish I could say I had not been betrayed
But it would not be so
I wish I could say I had not been let down

But it would not be so
I wish I could say I had not been mistreated
But it would not be so
I wish I could say I had not been misrepresented
But it would not be so
I wish I could say I had not been ignored
But it would not be so
I wish I could say that I feel safe
But it would not be so
I wish I could say that all the myriad things we have done to raise genuine awareness of ME had been effective
But it would not be so
I wish I could say that there is a safe medical pathway for my illness
But it would not be so
I wish, how I wish, that I could say that people understand the difference between ME and CFS
But it would not be so.
I wish I could say there is reliable diagnosis
But it would not be so
And I really wish I could say that there is a cohesive representation of my illness
But it just would no longer be so
I wish I could say with certainty that everyone with a diagnosis of ME actually has it
But the truth is that it is so misdiagnosed, misrepresented, misunderstood
That it horrifyingly, sadly, unacceptably, would just not be so.
I wish I could say that I had been adequately investigated

But it would still, decades on, not be so
I wish I could say I have adequate medical support
But it would not be so
I wish I could say that research purporting to be for ME is definitely looking at my illness
But it just would not be so
I wish I could say there is hope for the future
But it just would not be so
I wish I could say I have confidence in the charities supposed to be representing ME
But it just would not be so
I wish I could say the Government is doing all it can to ensure accurate diagnosis and to provide a biomedical treatment pathway for ME
But it just would not be so
I wish I could say that the most severely ill people with ME are treated with medical respect and are at the forefront of medical research
But it just would not be so.
Shocking isn't it?
Or is it?

22
WHEN I CAN, WHEN I CAN'T, WHEN I MIGHT, BY LINDA CROWHURST

∽

'When I can, when I can't, when I might.' You might call this my mantra, for it has been the way I have had to live my life for over a quarter of a century now. It is an interminable, probably unimaginable, amount of time to suffer intensely and invisibly.

Before I totally physically collapsed and became unable to get out of bed, you might well have said my mantra was this:

'When I chose, when I will, when I do' or something similar.

Now none of that is possible.

> For the person living in off the scale pain continuously, repeatedly paralysed, disappearing from one's own thoughts, memories and ability to feel or move, massively hypersensitive to noise, light, perfume and movement, a new

understanding of your reality must be urgently sought and a safe way to manage within it must be created.

It takes time to learn and try to understand what is happening to you; the bizarre and unpredictable reactions of the body, the continual deteriorations and intensifying of symptoms that lead you to live, literally in a state of continuous suffering. Trial and error was our path. Being able to move or think in some moments, but not all, being able to tolerate someones presence, even someone you love and want to be with, in some moments, but not all, being able to get even the slightest physical care needs met, in some moments, but not all, is a puzzling and upsetting thing initially.

For this pattern of severe symptoms, leads to an inability to flow with anyone in normal time, in the normal way, in the normal environment.

The way to help must be figured out. It is not obvious. The way to cope with it, must be forged out of impossible moments. A different way of looking at yourself and the world must be found, one that is based on your new physical, cognitive, emotional and spiritual experience. A new awareness on every level must be discovered. Compassion for yourself and everyone else must be developed, for you truly live in a world that feels as if it has been turned on its head, yet no one else can see it or feel it as you do.

Over time then, we came to this basic understanding and awareness. Not all moments were equal, in turns of access, tolerability, possibility. We could not be with each other when we wanted, how we wanted, the way we wanted, if at all and we could do nothing together that we had previously loved or enjoyed. When we were able to be together, every sound, every movement, every action, every contact, conversation, expression of affection, had to be monitored, controlled, minimised, done in a specific, sensitive, careful, way only and even then it might be too much.

Yet the times when anything was possible or tolerable, were not obvious, were not predictable, were not reliable and did not last. Cruelly, the very moment I might feel I could manage something, would literally be the second before nothing was tolerable. Any intervention or interaction of the tiniest effort, would lead to indescribable negative impact, despite that being farthest from its intention.

In these circumstances, life feels like a constant, rollercoaster of inability, inaccessibility, torment and separation. However, over time I came to see the need for calm inner being, patience and the recognition that things could and might change, just for an instant perhaps or hopefully longer, become more possible, at some other moment than the terrible painful, paralysed, tormented moment that I was stuck in, that seemed as if they would consume me totally. It is a terrible place to be in to be hungry, to need the toilet, to be screaming internally with pain, to lose your thoughts and your memory and not be able to get any of your basic needs met to alleviate the situation.

Because of this, I learned that in some moments, with certain levels of symptom intensity and specificity, absolutely nothing was bearable and for either of us to try to ignore that reality was dangerous and deteriorative. I also learned that there might be moments when I felt I needed something, wanted to try and yet still I could not tolerate the help required to aid me and then there were other moments when I thought I might manage, yet still I could not, though occasionally the opposite might be true.

Most moments I have to wait, still, all these decades later. Yet just occasionally something will shift, unbidden, uncontrolled, unpredictable, unexpected yet hoped for, yet nevertheless creates a possibility of movement, partial access, help to achieve something, not huge things in the way of the ordinary life, yet huge in a life shredded by emptying paralysis, intense hypersensitivity and continual bouts of completely numb, blank, lost cognitive ability.

We learned that certain times might be better than others, there might be more likelihood of success. We have also tried to look for patterns that might free us to understand my reality and my reactions better.

What I have learned is this.

Not every moment will be lost to everything, if only I can wait for and find the right moment.

So my mantra helps me to remember that there might be a moment just round the corner when things might feel more tolerable or possible and that helps me get through the impossibility of most of my life.

Sometimes I will feel or want to try something. It may or may not be possible.

And then just occasionally, in very simple ways, in an extremely limited, seemingly bizarre life, a wonderful thing happens; I want something and I can have it, just for a moment and those moments are the best.

23

PART TWO: KEY SYMPTOMS OF SEVERE AND VERY SEVERE ME

HERE WE TRY AND gain more understanding of Severe and Very Severe ME in terms of the underlying symptom experience. The symptoms are so extreme and so devastating that it takes highly skilled care to ensure people get their needs met.

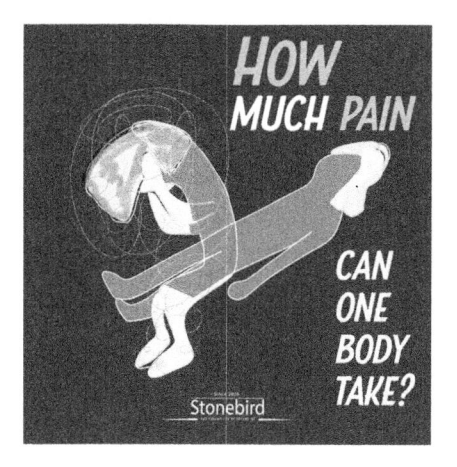

There is a great need to better understand the individual experience that people with a Severe ME/Very Severe diagnosis are going through.

24

HOW DO YOU CONVEY HOW VERY ILL YOU ARE?

Poetry is an immediate way to express things not so easily articulated in prose or direct speech. We have both been poets since our childhood expressing our deepest feelings. The more ill Linda has become and the more profoundly disabled she is, the more in pain, the deeper the devastation of paralysis and suffering she experiences, the more she turn to poetry to try and express something of her experience so that others might gain some semblance of understanding and empathy.

∼

How do you convey how very ill you are,
When words seem to lose their meaning,
as the illness takes a tighter and tighter grip on you?
First you say, "I am ill."
Then you say, "I am very ill."

Then I am "seriously ill."
Then I am "severely ill."
Then I am "worse."
Then I am "very severely ill."
Then I am "profoundly affected."
You try to explain each symptom,
But how do you convey multi-level pain,
impacting with different sensations?
How do you convey it is somehow more complex,
    torturing, intense
Than anything you would know?
"Pain," I say. "Burning pain. Throbbing pain. Itching
    pain. Numb pain."
"Worsening pain."
"Screaming pain."
"Deterioration."
Then "more deterioration."
Then "worse deterioration."
"Agony, torment, torture, literally."
Then there is the hypersensitivity.
"Acute."
"Extreme."
"Unimaginable"
"Indescribable."
"Destroying."
"Minimising."
"Separating."
"Hurting."
"Harming."
"Paralysing."
"Raging."

"Rampant."
Then there is the brain fog, creating absolutely "zero" in your mind.
"Emptiness."
"Separation."
"Isolation."
The loss
Becomes a "void."
"A vacuum."
"Nothing."
"Empty nothing."
"Numbness."
"Blank."
But what does that feel like?
What does that look like?
How horrendous does it have to be
For people to "get it",
Then respond with genuine empathy?
Compassion?
Honesty?
Kindness?
Recognition?
Why, instead, am I left in this splendid isolation,
Forced upon me by profound, indescribable symptom desolation, without relief,
That simply is overlooked, denied, ignored, by most
Leaving me feeling like a pariah and a ghost
In my own life?
Feeling that no one actually recognises,
nor understands, in the normal world,
The sheer level of suffering,
That continues without letup,

For decades?
Leaving me feeling that there are simply no words,
To describe my reality
Because I ran out of them over twenty-five years ago.
Yet still, it carries on.

A SYMPTOM SEVERITY SCALE

∽

It has always been a great frustration for us, that people with Severe ME are often described in behavioural terms, rather than in terms of their physical disease experience. Further, people tend to assume a generalised level of illness experience, with a Severe ME or Very Severe diagnosis, yet each person has their own unique experience within that level.

No two people are exactly alike. Some have greater specific symptom experience than others. Some are unable to leave their bed. Others are unable to leave the house.

The assumption that one is somehow more ill or disabled than the other, may or may not be true, depending on the severity of symptom experience that is disabling them:

- Some will be able to go out occasionally, others will have to remain indoors
- Some may find partial relief through treatment or be

able to use partially protective aids, whilst others can tolerate no drugs or protective aids
- Some may have severe or profound levels of hypersensitivity, others not so much.

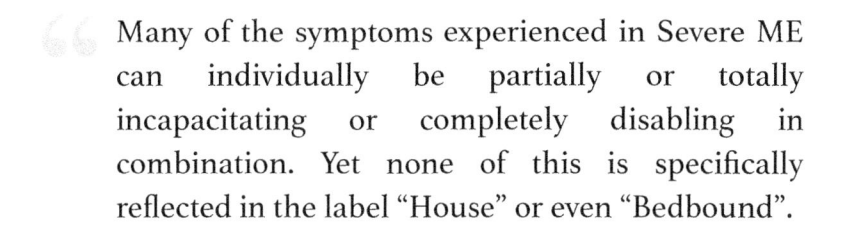

> Many of the symptoms experienced in Severe ME can individually be partially or totally incapacitating or completely disabling in combination. Yet none of this is specifically reflected in the label "House" or even "Bedbound".

Sensitive aware care needs to be honed skilfully to provide an individual approach. The carer going to an ME household may not understand the difference between clients, depending on which symptoms are more severe.

Health providers may not understand why some people diagnosed with Severe ME may be able with huge effort and aid, to attend hospital appointments whereas others may not be able to leave their home, travel or endure a hospital or clinic environment at all, even if help and assistance is available.

Some may attend meetings and speak on their own behalf. Others may have lost the power of speech altogether. Others still may need to be spoken for on behalf of them, with their permission. It really is a very individual thing. And it may also vary over time and in severity.

Two people may say they have light sensitivity, but they may not tolerate the same light exposure, similarly too with noise.

We feel Severe and Very Severe ME are better recognised by identifying the intensity of symptom experience. Without acknowledging the full range of symptoms, how can medical understanding and appropriate medical input ever be provided?

In order to create an individual understanding of each person's disability, it is very important to recognise that there is a range of ability and severity, even within the Severe/Very Severe ME category.

Not everyone will have the same symptoms, nor the same symptom experience and hypersensitivities, nor will they all have the same environmental challenges to deal with.

> There is a great need to better understand the individual experience that people with a Severe ME or Very Severe diagnosis are going through.

A much better disability scale, not so exclusively focused on behaviour, we suggest, needs developing.

Identifying a *Severity Scale* for each symptom would provide a much clearer, more detailed individual picture of what the person is experiencing and greatly aid understanding of how to help and interact more safely.

At long last, hypersensitivity levels would be recognised for the level of disability they specifically create in themselves or in conjunction to each other.

Hypersensitivities directly impact upon:

- how you interact
- how isolated you are
- how devastated you can be by people in your presence
- how you tolerate carer support
- how you need care to be provided to get the help you need in the right way at the right time.

A simple chart could help. Hypersensitivity severity could be ordered for each type as follows:

- **Absent**
- **Mild**
- **Moderate**
- **Severe**
- **Very Severe**
- **Profound**

For this purpose the person should always be the one identifying severity level.

Not everyone has hypersensitivities to the same degree or necessarily experiences them all at all. The level of severity may be constant or fluctuate.

You could determine which level of severity you have for each hypersensitivity, by using the following tentative descriptions as a rough guide:

- **Absent** = Not present
- **Mild** = Irritating, inconvenient, aware of
- **Moderate** = Irritating and painful, can be incapacitating
- **Severe** = Very painful and incapacitating
- **Very Severe** = Tormenting, isolating and considered unbearable
- **Profound** = Tortuous, completely disabling, totally isolating, intolerable, unimaginable.

Using a chart like this for light, noise, vibration, chemical, perfume, movement, motion, touch sensitivity or other symptoms too, could really help the person convey their needs better.

It could help the person present their own unique experience in a simple visual way.

It could help health providers better understand the specific issues facing people because of their individual and combined symptom impact.

For example, currently if you say ' I have a perfume or chemical sensitivity', you are left at the mercy of how aware a professional, friend or family member is, what they understand "chemical sensitivity" to mean and how willing they are to accommodate you.

Those two words do not convey the severity nor do they necessarily indicate how seriously chemical sensitivity must be taken.

Someone with moderate noise sensitivity and someone with profound noise sensitivity will both have noise sensitivity as their symptom, but will still experience noise very differently and need even greater care, in the latter case.

This really does need much better recognition, especially for those Very Severely affected, whose hypersensitivities may be off the scale.

Using symptom and hypersensitivity severity as opposed to behaviour to define disability levels would be a real change in emphasis. There needs to be much better recognition of the full symptom experience that people suffer, alongside a robust search for underlying physiology.

26

EXPERIENCE AND UNDERLYING SYMPTOMS

∼

THE SYMPTOMS THAT ONE experiences may all melt together into an overwhelming agony that is not easily defined or easily recognised an articulated. Symptoms may not be easy to separate out, rather the person may only be able to say what they cannot do or cannot tolerate, without knowing or understanding specifically why.

> Remember that symptoms have a cause and a pathology even when not identified as such and should be taken seriously and respected.

This is not a full list, just a few possibilities worth considering.
I can't think:
Cognitive impairments (impaired attention, memory and

reasoning) are among the most frequently reported and least investigated components of ME.

I can't understand:

Processing problems, brain fog, intermittent partial or complete memory loss, recurrent stupor or stroke-like episodes, tremors, aphasia, ataxia, dyscalculia (maths difficulty).

I can't tolerate noise:

Hyperacusis, loss of adaptability and worsening of symptoms with stress. Pain triggered by noise. Paralysis triggered by sound or vibration. Headache and or pain intensified or triggered, may be severe extreme. May affect confusion or disorientation. May have Tinnitus.

I can't speak:

Word, number and thought sequencing difficulties, difficulty with voice production, paraphasia – incorrect word selection, paralysis

I can't sleep:

Reversed sleep pattern disturbance, hypersomnia, vivid & disturbing dreams

I can't eat:

Food intolerances, difficulty with swallowing, choking, abdominal pains, problems with diarrhoea, swollen stomach

I can't sit up:

Muscle weakness, severe pain, palindromic arthropathies, dysautonomia

I can't walk:

Pain, muscle fatigue, paralysis, persisting dysequilibrium and ataxia, cardiac arrthmia, angina-like chest pain

I can't telephone:

Noise sensitivity, no energy, muscle weakness, loss of memory, concentration, intractable pain

I can't write:

Pain, weakness, numbness, parasthesia, cognitive impairment, agraphia (inability to locate the words for writing), neurological changes in motor skills (handwriting, coordination, vision)

I can't get to the toilet:
Muscle dysfunction and twitching/spasms, orthostatic intolerance, post-exertional muscle fatiguability, recurrent nausea and profound, incapacitating symptoms. Light-headedness and/or syncope (fainting), lower than normal blood volume, hypotension, hypoglycemia, cannot walk, cannot move.

I can't wash myself:
Poor coordination, pain in muscles, joints, head, back, limbs, chest and stomach, not enough energy, memory issues, unsafe standing, difficulty getting in and out of a bath or shower, cannot grip on safety rails, loss of feeling or sensation, dizziness

I can't stand up:
Orthostatic intolerance, muscle fatigue, weakness, difficulty with breathing, no energy, sudden attacks of breathlessness, dyspnoea, dizziness, painful or weak muscles and/or joints; the more severely affected are unable to stand unsupported for more than a few moments if at all and even then, may be completely unsafe.

I can't cook:
Transient paralysis, pain, cognitive dysfunction, confusion, disorientation, poor coordination and balance, dizziness or cognitive slowing, loss of fine motor skills, muscle weakness, loss of gross motor skill, numbness.

I can't read:
Dry eyes, pain, blurred and double vision, difficulty in focusing, swollen and painful, weak or paralysed eyelids, word

blindness, alexia (problems with reading), paralysis, cognitive difficulty with processing or understanding text.

Colour hurts my eyes:

Neuralgia, disorders of colour perception, photophobia, cognitive issues.

Touch hurts me:

Hyperesthesia, light touch can be acutely painful, pressure intolerable, continuous physical intense pain, including burning, throbbing, itching, stabbing, crawling, heightened by touch or pressure, neuralgia, muscle dysfunction.

People's energy affects me:

Severe lack of energy to cope with others presence, agnosia (the inability to process sensory information), impairment of concentration, difficulty with visual and aural comprehension, an exaggerated response to normal, to even small amounts of additional input, overstimulation, unable to interact two-way or respond to demand from others, other symptoms may be too extreme and require total attention to cope.

Light hurts me:

Photophobia, perceptual and sensory disturbances, spacial disorientation, abnormalities of sensation.

Food hurts me:

Food intolerance, IBS, problems with maldigestion or malabsorption of food, histamine intolerance, esophageal spasms, difficulty swallowing, throat muscle paralysis, gastroparesis, esophageal reflux, changes in taste and smell, bloating, abdominal pain, nausea, indigestion or vomiting.

27

DEALING WITH SYMPTOMS

~

ME is a well-documented, neurological disease acknowledged by the World Health Organisation. It is not a psychiatric illness.[1] The person you help is physically ill. [2]The needs may vary and the ability to communicate with you clearly may also vary.

The abilities of the person may vary throughout the day. You need to learn how the illness impacts specifically on the person you are helping. Each person may be different.

Main Symptoms you may come across:[3]

PAIN

There may be various sorts of pain[4] and odd sensations experienced. Pain may come and go or be constant or vary in intensity.[5] There may be no effective drugs available or tolerable to alleviate the pain; the person you help may just have to cope with the pain; no matter how bad.

There may be:

- burning
- throbbing
- crawling
- itching
- muscle pain
- skin pain
- joint pain
- all over body pain

The person in pain is very sensitive to touch and how you approach them to help may be key to success or failure; especially if they need physical assistance.

Head Pain

Head pain and headaches may be extreme and long lasting. They may go on for days or weeks at a time without relief. For some people they may be a permanent feature without relent. They my cause acute eye pain and may be left or right-sided. They may be completely incapacitating, making communication extremely difficult.

They may result in the person having to be incredibly still without any stimulation or noise, to try and cope. Decision making may be impossible at these times. There may be no effective pain relief available or tolerable.

Abdominal, Stomach and Menstrual pain

People may experience abdominal pain and stomach ache, which may be associated with IBS type symptoms, which adds to the general level of pain and discomfort.

> There may be other gastric issues causing pain that may need exploring, which is easier said than done in Severe ME, especially if you are too vulnerable and frail of health to attend hospital.

Body pain may also be associated with low cortisol[6] and it is important to check this out when body pain is an issue.

Menstrual pain may also be increased and more severe with ME, the impact of the hormonal shifts upon the body cannot be underestimated and can affect the level of symptom distress. Vaginal pain may an embarrassing pain that is difficult to talk about and not understood by the medical profession.(Robinson 2010)[7]

ME has been associated with early menopause, gynaecological problems and pelvic pain[8].

Vaginal pain may an embarrassing pain that is difficult to talk about and not understood by the medical profession. (Robinson 2010)[9]

A person with Severe ME for many years may also be fragile physically and be more likely to pull their ligaments and tendons, hurt their muscles and bump into things, fall over or be at risk of hurting themselves. Ehlers-Danlos Syndrome (EDS) [10]and Joint Hypermobility may be associated comorbid conditions.

The danger for somebody who experiences constant and chronic pain is the difficulty in identifying when something else, other than their ME is causing the pain. Always take new pain seriously and get it checked medically rather than just assume it is more of the same.

For the person suffering from long term total allover pain, there is something indescribably wonderful about getting unexpected pain relief and healing for a specific pain that they have had to endure, because it was in fact caused by something other than their ME and was treatable.

It is all too easy to think that everything is ME; it is important that the carer remains vigilant in this aspect, as well as the person.

VISUAL DISTURBANCE

[11]Vision may be disturbed in different ways.

Eyesight may seem like looking down a dark tunnel, muscles will not hold their focus, eyes may be dry, sore, itchy, swollen, may feel numb, burn, may not hold their tear film, may stare, may experience sharp pain from impact of light or effort of trying to move eyes or attempting to focus.

[12]The impact of visual disturbance may make reading extremely difficult, to impossible for the person with Severe ME; they may experience double letter vision, fuzzy sight, words may seem to move about or expand and contract. Lines may seem to shift about. It may be difficult to read columns or follow lines.

It may be possible to read a few words or paragraphs, but not whole pages or documents or books.

Visual disturbance in conjunction with cognitive dysfunction may mean that even if the person knows how to read, they may not be able to read, because they may not be able to comprehend the information.

Receiving and processing information can make reading difficult to impossible. Similarly writing may become difficult to impossible, even if a person can briefly hold a pen, if they are too visually disturbed or poorly coordinated to achieve it or struggling to comprehend what they see.

They may have difficulty coordinating vision, thought and function, it may be difficult to impossible to write on a line or to write on two consecutive lines or to write at all. Add fine motor control problems and writing may become impossible or illegible.

> Visual disturbance, in Severe ME, cannot be totally separated from cognition and motor control and physical dysfunction, as they all seem to have an impact upon each other, disabling communication, comprehension and expression for those who are particularly severely affected.

Even if the visual symptoms are not extreme the cognitive dysfunction may still make reading and writing limited to impossible.

Light sensitivity is a further barrier to communication and can cause eye pain and visual difficulties. Remember that any symptom can be exacerbated and made worse by environmental or post- exertional impact, so even the person who can barely manage something in one moment, may not be able to manage it in most or it may come and go unpredictably, or make them so ill it would be unwise to attempt.

Headache and eye pain may be closely linked, along with neck pain.

Transient, Periodic or Long term Paralysis

You may be surprised to find that the person you are helping has various degrees of paralysis in various parts of the body at varying times of the day and night:

- Sleep, for example may lead to overall body paralysis which may last several hours or longer
- Being in a stationary position following movement may also lead to transient paralysis

Therefore never assume that a person can do the same thing all the time. Always ask what help they need, unless they have told you they do not want you to speak to them whilst in this state. In that case you need to communicate with the person when they are more able to explain their needs. Or ask for written instructions as to how to help them if possible, in advance. Or ask that someone they know tells you what is needed.

Remember that a person who is paralysed may not be able to open their eyes, it does not necessarily mean that they are asleep:

- They may not be able to speak or call out
- They may have difficulties swallowing
- They may not be able to move their arms or legs or sit up or stand up without assistance
- Their pain may increase when in this state so do be aware
- Mobility will be extremely difficult depending on which parts of the body are paralysed. It could be left-sided paralysis or right -sided, partial or total
- They may be cognitively impacted after paralysis

PINS AND NEEDLES

This may not be like ordinary pins and needles that you shake off and it goes away:

- It may last a very long time or not go away all day or at all
- It may come and go
- It may be triggered by vibration ie sitting in a car

- Their body may go 'dead 'and be extremely difficult to get sensation back into
- They may experience pins and needles anywhere in the body and in unusual, unexpected places ie tongue, throat, ear, side of head, face, nose
- It may be a very unpleasant and painful experience

Muscle Spasms

These may be like fine tremors of the muscle, barely discernible or may be whole limb or even whole body spasms. They may be quickly over or continue for several hours. They can be very exhausting. They may be upsetting to observe especially when new to helping.

Noise Sensitivity (Hyperacusis)

This is a severely disabling symptom in its own right, causing acute difficulties with communication and being in the presence of other people. It makes going out into the world very challenging or even impossible.

You need to be aware that things you do without thinking or noises in the outside environment may be tormenting the person. These include things like :

- rustling a paper or plastic bag
- turning the page of a magazine or newspaper
- walking in the room
- noisy feet walking up or downstairs
- banging cupboard doors or drawers
- washing up
- tidying things away
- ringing bells
- sirens
- passing car engine

- running car engine
- letter box rattling
- dog barking
- doorbells or knocking at the door
- opening a tin
- opening or shutting a door
- eating a meal
- cutting something up on a plate
- telephone
- radio
- television
- music
- singing
- dancing
- a clock ticking
- speaking normally, even speaking in a whisper may be too loud

It requires great awareness on the part of the person helping someone who suffers from noise sensitivity. Sound reducing aids such as noise reducing curtains and glazing may be helpful.

LIGHT SENSITIVITY (PHOTOPHOBIA) AND VISUAL ACUITY

[13]The person with light sensitivity or photophobia may have it to varying degrees.

- It may be that the person needs to use dark glasses even in normal daylight
- They may need to have the curtains pulled during the day and they may need to hide under the bed clothes if you need to put a light on in order to help them or use some form of eye mask

- They may lie all day with their eyes covered not being able to bear any light
- They may cope with subdued lighting at night but not cope with the main light being switched on

Light can cause physical pain to people with this symptom. You may need to negotiate with them how best to help them, if you need a light on to see something they need. You need to work in partnership on this.

Eyesight may be affected and reading becomes difficult to impossible, due to the eye muscles not holding their focus. There may be double letter vision, letters may appear to dance around the page. It may be difficult to follow lines or columns. Don't just assume that reading is easy or possible.

Irritation[14]

The person with Severe/Very Severe ME may become irritated very quickly by noise or your voice or other sources of stress, because they are overstimulated. This can happen very quickly and may not be easy to judge.

You need to understand that the person may be extremely hypersensitive to many stimuli and you may need to stop speaking or leave the room or wait till the person has calmed again. This is something you need to be aware of and not take personally. You need to develop awareness of things you do that might aggravate the situation, so that you can try to avoid exacerbating the symptom.

Sleep Disturbance

The person may have insomnia and be unable to sleep nights on end or may have an altered sleep pattern, not sleeping till the early hours of the morning and sleeping way into the afternoon. Despite difficulties getting to sleep, the person may then experience difficulty waking up or may keep falling back into further bouts of sleep without being able to stay awake. They might feel like their body or mind has not woken up all day.

This could have a big impact upon when you are needed to help the person. The times people need help may vary considerably. The help they need may not fit into the normal pattern of everyday life. For example, breakfast may be eaten at lunchtime. Timings may be skewed because of this.

PENE, POST-EXERTIONAL NEURO-IMMUNE EXHAUSTION

[15]Any activity, mental or physical, even as slight as moving a limb, can lead to a worsening of symptoms and extreme exhaustion, that may mean muscles will not function, pain may increase dramatically and the person may feel more ill. This is called Post-Exertional Neuro-Immune Exhaustion. It is not like ordinary tiredness or fatigue.

The post-exertional exhaustion may be long lasting and may not even manifest for several days to several weeks after the particular action. This makes it very difficult to know what is impacting upon the person, it is also incredibly difficult to determine how much is too much, especially for the more severely ill.

For the person very severely affected, the minimal exertion for basic living can be too much; even if, from an outside view, they appear to have done little to nothing, it still may have a post-exertional affect.

It is absolutely imperative to understand the level of illness and disability of the person you are trying to help so that you do not inadvertently cause the person to do more than they can manage, by, for example, asking them a question or talking too long.

PENE is considered to be the hallmark of ME.

HEAT/COLD INTOLERANCE

There may be issues of temperature dysregulation[16]. They may exhibit periods of overheating and/or sweating profusely followed by bouts of feeling freezing cold. Sitting or lying still too long may exacerbate this as might paralysis for those who experience it.

There may be an intolerance to hot or cold temperatures. Heat can make the person feel more ill, cold can make the person more unable to move. They may feel shivery.

> " I fluctuate throughout the day from being so cold I cannot get warm, my nose and face feel like ice, my bones feel frozen to the core, then it will shift and I am sweating profusely and feel really hot. It is very exhausting. At these times there is also a risk of my skin breaking down on my face. I continually need to take clothes off when too hot, to put extra clothes on and needing blankets and other sources of warmth when too cold".

This has an implication for care, as it is not easy to continually change clothing or provide support with further need to wash or shower. Touch and pressure sensitive along with partial or total temporary paralysis or a complete lack of energy to deal with it all, may be an added stress. It means extra work for the carer and possibly more washing and expense."

NAUSEA

Nausea may be a permanent or near permanent feature and the person may also have fits of vomiting. Feeling sick will again have a huge impact on appetite, ability to cope, eating habits and generally feeling unwell.

COGNITIVE DIFFICULTIES

The person with Severe ME or Very Severe ME is likely to

have cognitive difficulties. This may be variable or constant. It may develop over time.

[17]It may cause problems with communication as their brain can have huge difficulties in receiving, processing and therefore understanding information

- It may feel to the person as if their mind has shut down, they may describe this as "brain fog". They may not be able to follow details or respond to questions or access memory or information.

Persistence with questioning or talking may lead to aggravation and worsening of symptoms. Even if someone can cope with a short conversation, they may be unable later to do the same again.

It may make reading, using the telephone, watching television, listening to the radio, having 2-way conversations, very difficult, if not impossible to do.

There may be a better time of day when the symptoms ease slightly and the person can better express their needs or think more clearly.

NUMBNESS

A person diagnosed with Severe or Very Severe ME may have a numb body. This again may vary in degree or come and go. A numb body means the person cannot feel properly. They may not be able to tell accurately the temperature of hot water or hot surfaces such as a cooker or heater. They may have less body awareness. They may fall easily. They may be at risk of burning themselves on i.e. a hot plate or a hot water bottle or in a bath or shower. These are important things for you to know, so that you can help a person safely.

DIZZINESS

A person may be dizzy at various times of day or when doing various things, such as moving from lying to sitting or sitting to standing. They may even be dizzy lying down flat. This is important for you to know, especially if you are physically assisting someone with these actions. Dizziness is not something obvious externally until someone stumbles or falls. Knowledge should help avoidance.

FOOD SENSITIVITY

Food sensitivity is a complex issue in ME. Sensitivity to foodstuffs [18] is one of the possible "immune, gastro-intestinal & genitourinary impairments" used for ME diagnosis, according to the 2011 ICC Criteria. [19]

My wife has been dogged with dietary issues, all the years she has had ME, resulting in difficulties eating dairy, wheat, refined sugar, oils, soya, gluten, carbohydrates. She has suffered continuing gastric issues, breathing difficulties and increased mucus, acid reflux, to distressing levels, impacting upon her whole life. The gastric issues in ME should not be underestimated or dismissed. They can be extremely debilitating and lead to severe weight loss.

It has been very difficult indeed trying to work out what is safe to eat. There have been years of struggling with massive weight loss. It has been very hard to find reliable professional advice to help us understand what is going physically wrong. We now believe there may have been some impact of histamine intolerance and there may have been Mast Cell involvement.

[20] We found food combining particularly helpful in trying to improve digestion.

We have been helped greatly by the *Cooking Without* [21] series of cookbooks by Barbara Cousins; a life-saver. Not only are the recipes free from ingredients that cause difficulties, they taste delicious to us and within such a stark context bring joy back into eating. They also seem to be infinitely adaptable, even if you omit or do not have to hand any particular ingredient.

It is too easy to describe the person with severe gastric issues, as just needing motivation to eat, without understanding the suffering they experience.

My wife's post-nasal mucus, for example, might not sound that serious, unless you look at it within the context of the impact upon her breathing, her gut, her muscles, her energy levels, her swallowing difficulties.

People need a balanced diet for vitamins, minerals and energy; having to give up whole food categories, is not easy. Food sensitivity and difficulty digesting food can so easily be misinterpreted without genuine understanding and knowledge of ME. There are also the issues of chewing and swallowing difficulties and possible gastroparesis to consider.

This is why it is so dangerous for people with ME, all the time the Health Service does not provide adequate and essential biomedical support from accurately informed ME practitioners, who can understand and look at the whole picture, not just a single symptom. Some people may need a Nasogastric tube or other interventions. It is a very serious issue. (Speight 2020)

> In Severe ME food sensitivity can lead to death. A dear friend eventually found eating impossible because of the excruciating pain caused by increasing sensitivity to more and more foods; eventually she could not tolerate any food and died from ME. She is not the only one we have known.

CARDIOVASCULAR DYSFUNCTION.

Cardiovascular dysfunction, with associated autonomic

nervous system dysfunction, including Chronic Orthostatic Intolerance; the inability to maintain a standing position and postural orthostatic tachycardia syndrome (POTS), extreme pallor, intestinal or bladder disturbances, has long been proposed as part of the ME disease process.

Cardiovascular dysfunction in ME patients has been well documented for many years, even so there has been little formal research on heart abnormalities in ME.

∼

SOME DAYS I am overwhelmed by the severity of my wife's symptoms, sometimes I look at her, with my heart breaking and full of fear.

---

1. For decades a powerful psychiatric lobby has wrongly asserted that there are no physical signs of disease and there is no pathology causing the patients' symptoms, and that because patients are merely "hypervigilant" to "normal bodily sensations", the illness should be managed by behavioural interventions to "reverse" patients' "mis-perceptions".(Hooper 2012) https://me-ireland.org/hooper.htm
2. ME is a disease where patients are more functionally impaired than those suffering from diabetes, heart failure and kidney disease, yet it has been sorely neglected by government health agencies.

    In 2012 the Consensus Panel, a group of doctors with over 500 collective years experience of studying and treating more than 50,000 people with ME, issued a one stop, user-friendly reference known as the Primer, (Carruthers B et al 2012) that specifically targets primary care physicians and specialists in internal medicine. It very strongly affirms that ME is not CFS and outlines many underlying biological abnormalities that are present more often in patients with ME. https://pubmed.ncbi.nlm.nih.gov/21777306/
3. In a survey I conducted of people diagnosed with Severe ME(n=21) , 71% of respondents reported that they experience 20 or more severe autonomic, endocrine, neurological and immune system manifestations :

    85% of respondents reported headache/pain.

Swallowing difficulties were experienced by over half (52%) the people surveyed

62% had noise sensitivity issues

67% had difficulty processing information

48% had unrefreshing sleep

66% had transient paralysis

85% had numbness

62% had photophobia

80% had perceptual/sensory disturbances

76% had heat/cold intolerances

48% had speech difficulties

33% had spasms

Each of these is a serious physical symptom in its own right. People with Severe and Very Severe ME experience multiple symptoms, all impacting upon each other causing serious disruption to physical functioning and resulting in severe disability.

Crowhurst G (2005) **One of the biggest medical scandals in history: a survey of those most severely affected by ME/CFS. Submission to the Parliamentary Inquiry into progress in the scientific research of M.E., by the 25% Severe ME Group** https://stonebird.co.uk/gibson.doc

4. There are various possible causes of pain in ME:
   - **Inflammatory cytokines**
   - **Bacterial neurotoxins**
   - **Nitrogenoxide** and other substances.
   - **Problem with the opiate receptors.**
   - **Poor delivery of oxygen to the organs**
   - **Mitochondrial dysfunction.**
   - **Ganglionitis**

   (De Meirleir, (2012) **Wetenschap voor Patiënten, Seminar 5: ME and Pain Web Seminar broadcast on november 30th, 2012** ME/cvs Vereniging, http://www.me- cvsvereniging.nl/)

5. Between 84% and 94% of ME patients, in research studies, report some degree of muscle or joint pain. (Breakthrough ME Research UK, Spring 2011 https://www.meresearch.org.uk/wp-content/uploads/2012/10/Breakthrough_Spring2011.pdf).

6. Most ME studies have found low morning salivary cortisol levels. Johnson C (2020) **Could Neuroinflammation Be Triggering the Cortisol Issues in ME/CFS and Fibromyalgia?** https://www.healthrising.org/blog/2020/06/18/cortisol-fibromyalgia-chronic-fatigue-syndrome-neuroinflammation/

7. Robinson S (2010) **Gynecological Concerns In ME/CFS Women** http://www.fightingfatigue.org/?p=8287

8. ME Research UK (2015) **Increased gynaecological problems** https://www.meresearch.org.uk/gynaecological-problems/

9. Robinson S (2010) **Gynecological Concerns In ME/CFS Women** http://www.fightingfatigue.org/?p=8287
10. Some people with ME likely have Ehlers-Danlos Syndrome Hypermobility Spectrum Disorder that has not been identified. Hakim et al (2019) CHRONIC FATIGUE IN EHLERS-DANLOS SYNDROME HYPERMOBILE TYPE AND HYPERMOBILITY SPECTRUM DISORDER (FOR NON-EXPERTS) https://www.ehlers-danlos.com/2017-eds-classification-non-experts/chronic-fatigue-ehlers-danlos-syndrome-hypermobile-type/
11. Visual symptoms are commonly reported in a range of neurological diseases, such as Alzheimer's and MS. They are also reported by people with M.E. ME Association (2018) Summary Research Review: Visual Impairment in M.E. https://meassociation.org.uk/wp-content/uploads/MEA-Summary-Research-Review-Visual-Impairment-in-M.E.-05.03.18.pdf
12. Eye symptoms are a concern to many people with ME; patients report sensitivity to light and dullness of vision to be significant problems. ME Research (2012) **Assessment of visual function in ME/CFS**
    http://www.meresearch.org.uk/wp-content/uploads/2012/10/Breakthrough_Spring2012.pdf
13. LIGHT SENSITIVITY IS ALSO known as photophobia. It can vary in the degree that different people experience it. For some it is a profound and beyond agonising symptom. How natural is it to just switch on the light, without thinking?

    But how do you help someone in the dark who is hurt by and who cannot bear light, for the extreme pain it causes?

    Not everyone can tolerate dark glasses or eye masks to try and cut down or block out light. Have you ever experienced what it is like, sitting indoors, the beautiful day outside calling to you, in agony, with the heaviest curtains you could get, tightly shut against the sunlight? Only the thickest, darkest curtains, tightly pulled will help. No chink of light must be left filtering through.

    Unexpected light exposure can cause such unnecessary suffering and unimaginable pain.

    As in all areas of care a profoundly aware, sensitive, creative, gentle approach, working together with the person to try and understand the needs, both of carer and person needing care, is required at ALL times. Light Sensitivity in Severe/Very Severe ME: a seriously challenging symptom, with no easy answers or explanations.
14. Symptoms may worsen with stress. This, said the late Dr Dowsett, who personally advised us to cut down on stress as much as possible, probably "arises from injury to the brain stem which normally controls the production of cortisol (a steroid required for stress control) via the hypothalamus, pituitary and adrenal glands. In the absence of an efficient response, even minor stress can cause catastrophic collapse in these

patients. NB. Because of the many and varied symptoms arising from encephalitic damage to the brain, all symptoms reported, however bizarre they may seem, must be taken as possible evidence of organic disease." Dowsett, Elizabeth (2001) THE LATE EFFECTS OF ME Can they be distinguished from the Post-polio syndrome? http://wames.org.uk/cms-english/wp-content/uploads/2012/04/Dowsett-THE-LATE-EFFECTS-OF-ME.pdf

15. For an excellent overview of PENE, also known as Post Exertional Malaise (PEM) please see this ME Association summary: https://meassociation.org.uk/wp-content/uploads/MEA-Research-Review-Assessing-PEM-in-MECFS-25.03.19.pdf
16. Heat and cold intolerance are common symptoms of ME and are recognised in the Canadian Consensus Criteria as a neuroendocrine symptom. ME-Pedia https://me-pedia.org/wiki/Body_temperature
17. Cognitive dysfunction is a very characteristic feature of ME. (ME Association (2019) https://meassociation.org.uk/2019/04/new-leaflet-from-the-me-association-cognitive-dysfunction-also-known-as-brain-fog-04-april-2019/)
18. ME Research UK (2016) **Milk protein intolerance** https://www.meresearch.org.uk/milk-intolerance/
19. Carruthers et al (2011) **Myalgic encephalomyelitis: International Consensus Criteria** https://www.ncbi.nlm.nih.gov/pmc/articles/PMC3427890/
20. The hypothesis that mast cells in the hypothalamus, triggered by environmental, neuroimmune, pathogenic or stress, activate microglia cells and disrupt normal homeostasis. Theoharides T (2018) **Extracellular vesicles from ME/CFS Patients and their effect on human mast cells and microglia mediators secretion.** https://solvecfs.org/theoharis-theoharides/

    According to Dr Nigel Speight Mast Cell Activation Disorder has probably been responsible for some actual fatalities. Speight N (2020) **Severe ME in Children** https://www.mdpi.com/2227-9032/8/3/211/htm
21. Cousins B (2000) **Cooking Without: All recipes free from added gluten, sugar, dairy produce, yeast, salt and saturated fat.** Harper Thomsons

28

ISSUES OF NOISE, LIGHT, TOUCH, CHEMICAL AND MOVEMENT SENSITIVITY IN SEVERE AND VERY SEVERE ME

∼

FOR THE PERSON LIVING with Severe/ Very Severe ME the environment, moment by moment, is likely to be a torment; the person helping them can increase, unintentionally, that torment through lack of awareness and sensitivity.

It can be extremely difficult for someone with Severe or Very Severe ME to get their needs met in a safe and caring way, when their acute and profound levels of hypersensitivity are invisible. They are so outside of most people's ordinary experience, that they are particularly hard to imagine.

> Carers need to find out which sensitivities a person has, what level of sensitivity they are, whether they are variable, constant and then work in a way that minimises daily exposure and impact.

One very small wrong intervention on the part of a carer can have dramatic and long lasting impact, causing indescribable suffering. It is a very serious issue, one that takes great commitment to try and comprehend.

Because communication is so complex in Severe and Very Severe ME, a verbal response is not always possible or for some, never possible.

> Your understanding of the situation as someone providing care, is vital, so that one mistake does not become many.

Noise sensitivity - Hyperacusis

Each person will be hypersensitive in different ways, one person may tolerate something that would destroy another. You need to understand that because you may have helped one person with ME, every person will not be exactly the same. Never assume you know anything or everything.

Here are some things not to do around or near someone who is noise sensitive, without first checking absolutely that the person can tolerate it occasionally, at all, or with limitations. Never ignore instructions.

ALWAYS DO WHAT IS ASKED, NOTHING MORE, NOTHING LESS. MORE CAN CAUSE UNEXPECTED, UNPREDICTABLE NOISE. LESS WILL NOT SUFFICE.

Do not do these things near the person unless they say they can tolerate it or unless the person is definitely out of hearing range:

- Do not shout

- Do not knock
- Do not bang things
- Do not cut things up, especially food, on a plate or hard surface
- Do not talk
- Do not drill
- Do not dig
- Do not mow the lawn
- Do not put the washing machine on
- Do not hoover
- Do not speak on the phone
- Do not let anyone in the house, including you, stomp on the stairs or the floor above the person
- Do not listen to music through headphones, not realising noise still leaks out and still causes harm
- Do not turn the radio or tv on, even in a different part of the house
- Do not boil a kettle
- Do not sweep or brush the floor
- Do not turn the tap on and especially leave it running
- Do not scratch your head or rub your face or hands together
- Do not cough in the room, if it can be avoided
- Do not sneeze or sniff, if it can be avoided
- Do not laugh
- Do not breathe heavily or too close
- Do not shower/run a bath that can be heard
- Do not wear clothes that rustle
- Do not flush the toilet whilst the person is there
- Do not run a car engine
- Do not open/shut a door

- Do not forget to shut a door so it bangs
- Do not open or shut a cupboard
- Do not wear noisy jewellery that clangs or clanks together
- Do not whistle
- Do not chat to a neighbour outside the window or at the door
- Do not leave a window open for noise to waft in unless expressly asked to
- Do not tap on a computer keyboard or tablet screen or use the printer, if it can be heard
- Do not open the mail, letters and parcels without agreement
- Do not do the washing up if it will be heard
- Do not read a newspaper that will rustle when you turn the pages
- Do not turn the page of a book
- Do not put things down on noisy surfaces or on any surface noisily
- Do not walk loudly in outdoor shoes
- Do not turn things on and off without awareness
- Do not eat near the person so that they can hear
- Do not pour a drink
- Do not play a musical instrument
- Do not wear a ticking watch
- Do not talk to yourself out loud
- Do not make any noise without warning
- Do not clap or tap hands or feet
- Do not leave mobile phone ringer on.
- Do not be uptight or angry or loud in your voice tone
- Do not yawn noisily

- Do not fidget
- Do not clank things together
- Do not write on a surface
- Do not switch things on or off that make a click
- Do not use your computer or tablet nearby or make any noise that can be irritating or indescribably tormenting
- Do not prepare food without taking precautions to avoid noise exposure
- Do not cook except in an agreed way and at an agreed time
- Do not move about the room unnecessarily or at all
- Do not do something if it is clearly causing pain and upset
- Do not make a noise repeatedly
- Do not move anything without agreement

> It is only when you stop and think about all these daily ordinary things that you do without thinking, that you begin to realise what a dangerous and tormenting world the person with severe to profound hyperacusis lives in.

They are hurt and harmed by the ordinary or even the quiet. As a result, how very hard it is to help the person and sustain contact and engage with the person without causing serious distress and harm. How very difficult it is to offer care in an appropriate and aware manner and maintain relationships.

> Even if you do not understand fully, still you need to accept and respect the person's reality or harm will follow.

Any noise can cause instant partial or total paralysis, for someone with profound Hyperacusis or may trigger:

- body shaking then paralysis
- skin going numb
- speech becoming impossible
- eyes staring
- guts tremoring
- muscles turning to jelly and collapsing
- pain intensifying everywhere
- pain from light increasing
- vision diminishing
- eyes staring
- swallowing becoming difficult
- overwhelming nausea
- shallow breathing
- hot sweats
- freezing extremities
- head and neck inflammation
- intense head pain
- face becoming palsied
- tongue going numb
- muscles throbbing, burning, itching, screaming with pain skin crawling with indescribable sensations
- energy instantly draining away
- all thought blanked out

Nothing is possible, contact is unbearable, communication unachievable. Noise sensitivity increases and lasts well after the noise has gone.

Unfortunately noise sensitivity, a torment in itself, does not just stand alone, but links in with other symptoms, increasing them too. Basically any noise, even a seemingly quiet noise to you, can still be a torment and a harm leading to worsening deterioration of symptoms and illness experience.

Noise can hurt or be so painful and destructive that it can cause paralysis, muscle spasms, cognitive confusion, severely worsening cognitive dysfunction, making the experience a literal torture where even the sound of breathing or whispering will be a nightmare for the person to experience.

For the most profoundly affected, noise, even a slight noise that you might not even notice or describe as noise or might accidentally or unintentionally make, can be so harmful that it is utterly traumatic and dangerous. It is not just the loud noise that causes problems. It may be certain sorts of noise, like voice tone or cutlery or the slightest click.

It is hard to truly comprehend the impact or register, even, what level of noise you are making, as infinitesimally small noises can hurt and trigger a devastating response if they are the wrong sound at the wrong moment, as much as large and repeated or constant sounds can.

Exposure to noise, especially loud and continuous noise can be inexplicably painful and cause lasting damage. The life of such a person can be an ongoing noise nightmare that makes every aspect of life inaccessible or indescribably difficult to tolerate and experience.

It is not just the sound itself that can hurt and be unbearable, but in the most sensitive people, the vibration itself can cause massive physical assault and cause unbearable muscle tremor and whole body spasms and whole or partial body paralysis, numbness and loss of proprioception. It is very serious and cannot be underestimated, down played, trivialised or ignored, nor the person expected to somehow get over it or 'pull themselves together.'

> Every sound, loud and small can feel as if the person is being repeatedly kicked in the head or pummelled all over their body or hit in the guts or worse.

Unfortunately living in the ordinary world, things make noise, even when trying to be quiet. It then becomes a complex dance between action and non-action, between leaving things however long they take or trying to figure out a way to avoid the noise or lessen its impact.

Some people may chose to wear ear plugs or ear defenders, others however cannot do so due to touch and pressure sensitivity. The daily living experience is particularly horrendous for them, especially if noise is unavoidable or noise issues ignored or forgotten or not addressed. Isolation, avoidance and protection are then, sadly, central strategies for living.

~

Light sensitivity - Photophobia

You might need to work out with the person how you can safely meet their need without exposing them to light.

This is a complex issue especially for the most severely affected and the importance of understanding the implications of ignoring or forgetting to respect this seriously disabling and invisible symptom, cannot be over emphasised.

Light is so much a part of the every day that it may be hard to imagine how much extreme pain it can cause to a person with very severe or profound light sensitivity.

Light Sensitivity can trigger muscle shaking, seizures, intense head, eye and body pain, increased inflammation, nausea, vomiting, paralysis, irritability, total deterioration of other symptoms and justified upset. The after impact of unexpected exposure can last for hours, days, weeks; can be indescribably damaging.

Here are some things not to do around or near someone who is light sensitive, without checking absolutely that the person can tolerate it either occasionally or with limitations.

DO NOT:

- Do not switch on the light for your own need
- Do not change the light bulb to a different strength
- Do not open the curtains even a centimetre to let in light so you can see, without agreement
- Do not leave the door ajar to let in light
- Do not forget to have a spare pair of dark sunglasses available in case they get broken
- Do not switch on the TV screen unexpectedly
- Do not switch on the computer screen unexpectedly
- Do not have the computer screen set on anything but the lowest brightness setting if tolerated
- Do not strike a match
- Do not flash a torch in the room and especially not at the person
- Do not ignore the pain and distress of acute photosensitivity
- Do not wear bright colours or brightly patterned clothes
- Do not wear sparkly things that shimmer
- Do not open the door and let in light unexpectedly
- Do not forget to close the curtains fully at night,

when it is dark, so that early morning light can penetrate and torment
- Do not forget to check that the person has whatever eye/body protection they need on and is able to tolerate and is prepared and in agreement, before exposing them to any light
- Do not shine a light directly at the person.
- Do not take a photograph with the flash on
- Do not move a person to another room without taking precautions to ensure that the person is still as light protected as possible and all issues have been thought through in advance
- Do not use a mobile phone with light screen pointed toward the person or in the room with the person
- Do not let someone unaware enter the room and cause pain and physical chaos through exposing the person to light unintentionally

Safety of the person is important alongside the health and safety issues of the person caring. This is a difficult issue to balance. Explore options that will enable you as a carer to help and support the person, whilst respecting the light sensitivity issue.

If you are care for someone, especially someone who has severe to profound light sensitivity, you must understand your impact upon the person. It is of absolute importance that you know what effect light will have upon the person.

You must know how to respond appropriately if the person is unexpectedly exposed to light. It is important to stay calm, centred, focused and not panic or do something else wrong.

. . .

Light exposure can result in:

- agonising eye pain
- head pain
- face pain
- throbbing burning, piercing pain
- extreme headache
- increased cognitive dysfunction
- light after-image lasting long after the source is gone
- shaking spasms
- nausea
- distress
- visual disturbance
- weakness
- paralysis
- irritability

∼

Touch Sensitivity - Hyperesthesia

The slightest touch wrongly made, can cause agony and deterioration and real distress or harm and last hours, days or longer, long after the contact has passed, for the person who has hyperesthesia is sensitive to physical contact and pressure or movement on the skin.

Understanding the implications of ignoring or forgetting to respect this seriously disabling and potentially invisible symptom is essential.

Here are some things not to do around or near someone who is touch sensitive, without checking absolutely that it is appropriate and the person can tolerate it occasionally, at all or with limitations or at certain times.

Personal contact may be necessary for performing intimate care but must always be agreed in advance, with the greatest possible respect and awareness of personal boundaries and appropriateness.

DO NOT:

- Do not make physical contact with the person without permission
- Do not reach out unexpectedly
- Do not move bedding without warning
- Do not lean against the person, rather let them lean against you
- Do not put pressure on the person's body while assisting them
- Do not try to lift them without warning nor try to lift them without their cooperation and preparation
- Do not hold them in the wrong way. Learn how to do this in the right way
- Do not try to help them without awareness
- Do not move limbs carelessly or without awareness to help with getting dressed or undressed
- Do not put clothes on the person that are too uncomfortable or tight or just not quite in the right place causing discomfort or agony
- Do not move the person without consent or in away they cannot tolerate
- Do not lean on or sit on the bed to talk or help
- Do not lean on or sit on the wheelchair to talk or help

- Do not do anything in a different order than the person is expecting
- Do not brush their hair without knowing how, when and if tolerable
- Do not put a tray or other object on top of the person or on their lap or on the bed clothes even
- Do not put anything on the bed, either on top of them or even beside them as the sensitivity can be so subtle it will hurt without being obvious

For visitors:

- Do not shake hands unless you know the person can tolerate the touch and pressure
- Do not hug the person, unless they say it is okay
- Do not kiss the person, unless safe to do so and wanted
- Do not hold hands with the person unless you know it is safe and acceptable
- Do not have any contact that you are uncertain is safe
- Do not pat the person on the back or arm affectionately unless you know it is tolerable and okay to do so

Someone with touch sensitivity needs to be helped in a gentle, compassionate, empathic and aware way. If touch is a necessary part of care, it is so important that the touch is gentle, compassionate, empathetic and rightly timed and appropriate.

Pain and hypersensitivity, however, can be so intense and constant that pain is unavoidable, even to meet the most basic minimal needs. So great care and precautions are required.

Never touch anyone diagnosed with Severe and Very Severe ME or unless you know it is tolerable and the contact is wanted and the moment is right.

For the affectionate person who reaches out in compassion and kindness to convey warmth and comfort, it may not come naturally to avoid touching or hugging a person, especially if they are in discomfort or distress.

However, natural instincts to reach out to comfort in the normal ways one would do, need to be altered in the presence of someone with touch hypersensitivity and severe pain, as the gentlest contact, meant lovingly, can still cause agony and deterioration and unbearable increase in symptoms.

TOUCH SENSITIVITY **in Very Severe ME:**

- causes agony on slightest contact
- has unbearable indescribable impact
- means pressure intensifies pain which already may be intolerable
- makes sitting, lying down intensely painful and/or impossible
- makes it difficult to tolerate physical assistance, even when needed, without causing deterioration of symptoms, can induce paralysis or shaking spasms, inflammation, nausea, blacking out, numbness, dizziness
- makes it hard to find suitable clothes that do not hurt or add pressure
- means the slightest accidental contact can really hurt the person and makes it hard to find suitable

materials or tolerate enough bedding to keep warm, without adding too much pressure
- makes it difficult to find comfortable, suitable, tolerable seating, mattresses, bedding etc.

∽

Multiple Chemical sensitivity - MCS

[1]Chemical sensitivity may be difficult to imagine or even notice for the person who does not have it, who lives generally in the world of perfumes and chemicals,[2] even enjoying the smells or becoming so accustomed to certain chemicals that they are simply not noticed.

Living with Multiple Chemical Sensitivity (MCS), people become isolated and alienated from the world and people around them. They also live tormented lives and are made extremely ill by exposure to chemicals and perfumes.

Some people with Severe ME develop MCS.

Here are some things not to do around someone who experiences MCS, unless you specifically have their agreement that they can tolerate it.

DO NOT:

- Do not wear perfumed products on the days you are helping and preferably never wear them, as they linger on clothing, hair etc. This includes deodorant, shampoo, aftershave, hand lotion, moisturisers as well as perfume itself
- Do not wear clothes washed in perfumed detergents. The person may be able to tolerate certain products

which hopefully you might choose to use your self to make life easier for you both
- Do not disregard the person's perfume and chemical sensitivity
- Do not use products to clean with, other than those specified as safe, by the person
- Do not buy any alternative product that has dangerous chemicals or intolerable perfumes as a substitute to please yourself or because something is unavailable. Always check ingredients
- Do not forget to ask the person for alternative products that they might accept, when shopping, in case the store has run out or order things online well in advance, to ensure that there are no problems with supply, in agreement with the person
- Do not leave windows open without being asked, as environmental chemicals can waft through the open window
- Do not expose the person to petrol or other fumes or bonfire smoke by leaving windows or doors open or by carrying the smell of them in on your clothing
- Do not clean without express permission, only perform cleaning tasks at the time the person can tolerate it, in the way they have asked you to do
- Do not expose the person to cleaning products that may have got onto your skin or clothes. Make sure you wash off all odours, as even if they may be acceptable or unnoticeable at a distance, close contact may still cause reactions
- Do not use herbicides or pesticides in the house or garden
- Do not use paint that is oil based and needs

chemicals to clean the brush unless expressly asked to by the person
- Do not use perfumed carpet cleaner
- Do not ignore the importance of being aware that the smell of certain drinks and certain foods may also trigger a bad reaction
- Do not sit down on any seats with perfumed products on you, as the smell may transfer and be impossible to get rid of and be dangerous or intolerable to the person. It can linger for many months
- Do not enter into any uncontaminated safe room if you think you may have chemicals or perfume on you. You may need to wash or change your clothes and shoes before entering or aiding a person with MCS
- Do not ignore instructions concerning food packaging when buying, storing and cooking and be aware of plastic bottles and containers. Packaging may have picked up perfume in the shop. If glass only has been stipulated, then stick with it. Plastic containers, utensils etc can be a danger to health with MCS
- Do not give the person water that has come from a potentially unsafe source such as a plastic bottle. Establish what is safe and what is tolerated before you begin to help the person
- Do not prepare food with different ingredients or unknown, untried sources, as their may be chemicals or flavourings etc that are harmful in them
- Do not suck strong smelling sweets

- Do not assume that natural, perfumed products, such as lavender oil, are tolerable because they are natural or organic. Always check with the person. Perfume free can still have an intolerable odour and impact

If you have MCS and you are exposed to chemicals and perfumes you cannot tolerate, they make you instantly react and become even more ill. They may trigger headache, nausea, rash, skin irritation, vomiting, muscle weakness, paralysis, numbness or other specific symptoms. It may affect breathing.

It is completely incapacitating to be chemically exposed. It can endanger your health and lead to you live a tormented and very isolated life.

You need to learn how to safely engage and work with someone with Severe or Very Severe ME and MCS. The ordinary things you take for granted will be a huge issue potentially. Carpets, bedding, new clothes, furniture, furnishings, decorating; all new products that have dyes and chemicals such as fire retardants, glues etc can cause allergy and/or sensitivity and may be intolerable and endanger health.

Exposure to chemicals and perfume can cause:

- burning skin and throat pain
- rashes
- nausea
- severe instant headache
- swallowing difficulties
- numb throat and tongue
- muscle weakness
- shaking
- indescribable collapse

- dizziness
- intense malaise
- burning eye and face pain
- massive deterioration; the after- effect goes on and on, with no relief.

~

Movement Sensitivity

Movement can be devastating to the person with this unusual sensitivity, whether this is movement past them, in front of them or physically moving the person while assisting them or even them moving themselves.

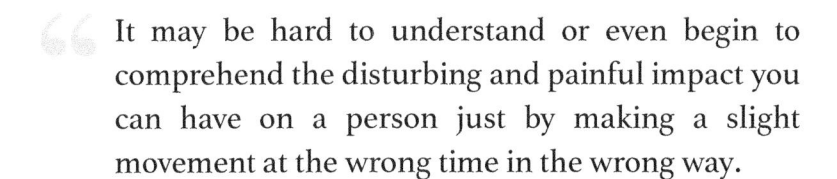

> It may be hard to understand or even begin to comprehend the disturbing and painful impact you can have on a person just by making a slight movement at the wrong time in the wrong way.

It is especially difficult, because we do a lot of things inadvertently and without awareness, such as move our hands to express ourselves or tap a toe or finger, scratch our head, wander about looking for things etc.

All these things we need to learn to control if possible. It does not necessarily come naturally, but the person helping someone with profound movement sensitivity needs to develop their own body awareness to a higher degree than is normal, so that they can move gracefully, peacefully and with consciousness, flowing with and being with the person, rather than irritating them further.

Here are some things not to do around or near someone who is Movement Sensitive, without checking absolutely that the person can tolerate it, whether occasionally, at all, or with limitations and how to accommodate helping them in the context of this complex Movement sensitivity, so that they can still get their needs met.

DO NOT:

- Do not make any fast movement at all that will cause irritation and deterioration of symptoms
- Do not scratch your head or body unnecessarily or if you have to, then indicate this first, to minimise the impact
- Do not gesticulate in the air
- Do not tap on things
- Do not type in view of the person unless expressly asked and agreed
- Do not push the person in a wheelchair, without letting them know that they are about to move so they can be prepared
- Do not push the person quickly in the wheelchair, unless asked to, as speed will increase the potential disturbance to the person as things move past them
- Do not pull the person backwards especially without warning. This can have a dramatic impact on the autonomic system, cause complete chaos in the head and be extremely disturbing, may cause nausea, dizziness, head pain, black out, irritation, distress, chaos in whole body, simply be intolerable and unbearable, without necessarily being able to adequately explain the experience or why it is so unbearable

- Do not move repeatedly past the person and especially not close to the person as they can actually experience the nearness as pain
- Do not move the person quickly while helping them unless this is necessary and with agreement. Movement can be painful, disorienting, disturbing, upsetting, deteriorative
- Do not walk with the person faster than they can tolerate or bear
- Do not take the person into crowded places or near groups of people if the person has to go out, for example, to a hospital appointment. The more people, the more movement and disturbance
- Do not drive faster than the person can cope with, if they can be in a vehicle at all, be aware that speed bumps can also cause distress as motion changes
- Do not drive on busy roads or at busy times of day if avoidable as vehicles driving fast towards the car can have a frightening impact, especially large and noisy vehicles
- Do not kick a ball or throw a ball or let a pet off the lead to run about back and forth in front of the person
- Do not hoist a person awkwardly or too quickly or without respect for their complex physical symptoms. To use a hoist or lift someone with movement sensitivity can be incredibly difficult to manage and for health and safety reasons requires training. Utmost respect and care is required to safely engage with and move the person. Make sure you understand how to do this properly. Make sure you stop and rest at intervals as required. Only move

a person in a way that they can cope with and with their cooperation

Obviously some movement is necessary. It is the how and when, that is important and when not to. It may be that familiar movements and routines will help and be better tolerated. It is unique to each person what they might tolerate or the best way to help them cope with your presence.

It is also about learning to be still in yourself and not doing extra movements that are unnecessary and risk irritation, exacerbation and deterioration. If you can learn to be present, aware and very still in yourself and graceful in your movement, there is a better chance of assisting productively.

～

THERE ARE no easy answers for these complex hypersensitivities. It may be trial and error. The important thing is to aim to flow and work with the person in partnership so that you do not cause further alienation and isolation for the person or harm, nor go away feeling you are a failure or that it is impossible to help the person.

You need to understand all the symptoms and how they interact together to impact the person. In reality they never work in isolation. The most important thing is to respect the person and know the way the illness manifests in them. Never disregard any medical information.

---

1. Multiple Chemical Sensitivity is officially recognised in the International Classification of Diseases, (ref: ICD 10: SGBV:3.1:code T78.4: Chemical Sensitivity Syndrome, Multiple)

2. Hooper et al (2001) postulated that there is convincing evidence that ME may be due in part to multiple chemical and/or biological exposures which have been shown to increase the permeability of the blood brain barrier (BBB), leading to a significant brain injury.

Hooper, M. & Montague S 2001. **Concerns about the forthcoming UK Chief medical officer's report on Myalgic Encephalomyelitis (ME) and Chronic Fatigue Syndrome (CFS) notably the intention to advise clinicians that only limited investigations are necessary.** https://www.academia.edu/32317688/Concerns_About_the_Forthcoming_Uk_Chief_Medical_Officers_Report_on_Myalgic_Encephalomyelitis_Me_and_Chronic_Fatigue_Syndrome_CFS_Notably_the_Intention_to_Advise_Clinicians_That_Only_Limited_Investigations_Are_Necessary

29

BITTER LANDS

I am in the bitter lands.
Everything here bites me.
The sound breaks me open.
The light burns me.
The movement destroys understanding,
Leaves me disoriented and blank.
Here I am washed out and emptied.
There is no feeling here
Except pain and empty numb being.
I am lost again in the twisted ground of paralysis.
My body is totally sucked out into nothingness.
My sense of myself is lost too.
My emotions ride a tsunami.
My mind has lost its direction.
My body has lost its boundaries,
As awareness floats away
And I feel like a swollen melon.
Nothing works,

Everything feels sick
And I am stuck on the outside
And dissipated on the inside,
Waiting for something inexplicable
To unpredictably shift
And restore some semblance
Of movement and life,
Once more.

30

THE PROBLEM OF PARALYSIS IN ME

∼

ME diagnosis is very poor in the UK. It relies on an inadequate, limited number of symptoms, seemingly plucked out of the air that bear little or no resemblance to the physical illness experienced by the most severely ill.

Paralysis is way off the list of accepted symptoms, despite it was recognised by the early pioneers of this serious neurological disease: Dr Ramsey, Dr Mowbray, Dr Betty Dowsett, as part of ME.

1

The problem of the name ME

Unfortunately ME has become dissociated from its original meaning and usage. No longer is the name Myalgic Encephalomyelitis used to depict a specific disease, linked with an Enterovirus.

It is now at best used as an umbrella term for a wide range

of conditions and illnesses which primarily focus on generalised fatigue in order to define them.

This means that the recognition of a symptom such as paralysis is harder to obtain and understand its connection.

If you say Polio, for example, paralysis is well known to be associated with it, though not everyone experienced it, there is a non-paralytic form. The Polio virus is an Enterovirus. The Link is still there potentially[2], but has been downgraded and almost lost now, due to a lack of recognition and promotion of Enterovirus as causative of ME.

[3]Nowadays there are a wide range of causes attributed to ME including psychological ones, which dangerously leads to the misinterpretation that any paralysis experienced in ME is likely to be hysteria or any of the other terminologies that psychiatry has come up with that deny the physical reality of it.

How will things ever change? How will the specific disease ever be uncovered and the people who have it, find a medical path that supports them correctly?

The problem of research

Research in ME does not, to our knowledge, focus on paralysis. We have tried over the decades to gain real interest and action on this issue to no real avail.

In 2013[4] we conducted our own survey to see how widespread paralysis is in people diagnosed with Severe ME. We received 46 responses which all confirmed varying degrees of transient awake or sleep paralysis.

In 2019 Jason et al [5] conducted a user-informed questionnaire on PEM for which 29.4% of respondents said that they had paralysis as part of PEM (Post-Exertional Malaise). That surely is enough people experiencing paralysis to raise concerns that the definitions and symptom identifiers for ME are inadequate? Or that the investigations are inadequate and any comorbid paralytic disease has not been identified or that the diagnosis is perhaps the wrong one?

Unless the underlying physiology of paralysis, in ME, is researched, how will anyone ever know why they are paralysed? How will they know what is the specific pathology underlying their paralysis if no one looks to see and no one compares people's experience and no one runs tests that might show up the why of paralysis, because it has already been mislabelled or ignored?

How will people who are paralysed, whether occasionally, repeatedly, daily, partially, totally or permanently get the medical input and right level of investigation, medical respect and answers, if few are willing to look, listen, learn, research, acknowledge, respond?

The lack of physiological explanation of paralysis in ME

Symptom experience without physiological explanation is open to misunderstanding, misinterpretation and mistreatment, however we have been able to find little information on the reason why paralysis occurs in ME.

If you weaken the Polio connection [6] and deny the enteroviral connection in ME, you have removed a specific pathology to reliably test for or provide explanation. You then have no baseline from which to progress your understanding. As paralysis was a key symptom originally, it could presumably have had proper medical input and concern, yet that medical specificity is not now there.

The apparent intent to eradicate ME as a neurological disease associated with Polio has been very effective.[7]

Paralysis leaves us asking:

- Is it caused by specific brain damage?
- Is it due to ganglionitis?
- Is it due to a channelopathy/ electrolyte imbalance?
- Is it genetic?
- Is it somehow linked to the HPA axis shifting, that is observed in ME?
- Is it due to Mitochondrial Dysfunction?
- Is it muscle paralysis?
- Could it have been drug induced, because without understanding the disease pathology, any treatment may be unsafe, if the impact is unknowable because the physiology has not been clearly identified?

These questions remain medically unclear and unanswered for us. Why is it sporadic in some, seemingly permanent in others, what might cause it to be transitory? We have no definite answers still for paralysis in those diagnosed with ME.

Do those who experience paralysis actually have ME at all? Have they been wrongly diagnosed? Or do they have a co-morbid condition that has been ignored due to the lack of biomedical understanding in ME currently? The lack of knowledge is unacceptable to us.

The experience of recurrent tortuous paralysis is overwhelming and dominating and indescribably painful and unjust. If anyone has answers, we would be really interested.

THE PROBLEM OF LANGUAGE AND DESCRIPTION.

One issue is the difficulty of identifying the specific experience each person has. The language is not necessarily there to describe the reality. The onslaught of symptoms makes it difficult to separate them out. What one might describe as fatigue, might actually be muscle weakness or muscle fatigue. What might be described as weakness and therefore inability to move may in fact be partial or total paralysis.

It is not necessarily easy to identify or articulate, also cognitive dysfunction may limit processing and language, therefore different people may describe the same symptom quite differently. Without the tests or even the recognition of paralysis as part of ME, there may be a higher prevalence than known.

Potential causes of paralysis

There are other diseases, better respected and treated with proper medical input. Here are a few:

- Periodic Paralysis
- Mitochondrial Disorder
- Hemiplegic Migraine
- Addison's Disease
- MELAS: Mitochondrial Encephalopathy, Lactic Acidosis and Stroke-like Episodes

We discovered that it is not only nerve damage that causes paralysis. Muscle dysfunction, electrolyte imbalance which can arise for different reasons, such as poor kidney function, aldosterone/renin imbalance, genetics and brain damage are but four examples.

The important thing is to realise that symptoms without the physiological explanations that should be attached, lead to misinterpretation, misunderstanding, potential mistreatment, neglect.

This unfortunately is where people with ME are left.

1. This tribute by Dr Charles Shepherd is a good overview of the work of Dr Betty Dowsett and Dr Ramsay https://meassociation.org.uk/2012/06/dr-betty-dowsett-1920-2012-consultant-microbiologist-who-championed-m-e/

    The late Dr James Mowbray was instrumental in developing the VP1 Test demonstrate the presence of viral protein in blood and brain tissue : *"we have been able to find a very large fraction of the ME patients have got an enterovirus antigen....Just because you find virus proteins in the blood, does that mean they are infected? Yes, it does....The virus is present in the intestine. It is also shown to be present in the muscle...What does it do in the muscle?....(It) does the thing that viruses usually do, they infect the cell and take over......"*. http://carersfight.blogspot.com/2016/05/why-separation-of-me-from-cfs-is-long.html

2. For more background please see Richard Bruno's comprehensive history: **Parallels between Post-Polio Fatigue and Chronic Fatigue Syndrome: A Common Pathophysiology?** https://www.papolionetwork.org/uploads/9/9/7/0/99704804/parallels_between_post-polio_fatigue_and_chronic_fatigue.pdf

3. For more on the Polio connection please see our paper on Channelopathy https://stonebird.co.uk/channelopathy/paralysis.htm

4. **Paralysis, a qualitative study of people with Severe Myalgic Encephalomyelitis** http://carersfight.blogspot.com/2013/08/paralysis-qualitative-study-of-people.html

5. Please see : https://www.ncbi.nlm.nih.gov/pmc/articles/PMC6468435/

6. Dr Betty Dowsett published a classic article comparing Post Polio syndrome and ME : http://wames.org.uk/cms-english/wp-content/uploads/2012/04/Dowsett-THE-LATE-EFFECTS-OF-ME.pdf

    Dr Byron Hyde's (2020) book "Understanding Myalgic Encephalomyelitis - The new polio and chronic fatigue syndromes. " discusses how ME, like paralytic polio, which in many ways mirrors ME, is a neurological injury.

7. Psychiatry has spent the last 60 years spreading the untruth that Myalgic Encephalomyelitis (ME), a WHO G93.10.3 classified neurological disease, is a mental health disorder. Tragically, psychiatry has been allowed to dominate social, health and welfare policy in the UK, for decades on end. For much more information on this please see my free eBook *Straightjacketed By Empty Air* : https://stonebird.co.uk/emptyair/sj.pdf

31

WHAT DOES PARALYSIS FEEL LIKE?

∽

It depends to an extent on the trigger.

Sleep is a constant trigger. Every sleep brings severe long lasting paralysis that takes many hours to minimally break free from. Every further sleep becomes a horrendous worsening nightmare from which I cannot escape, as it grips me deeper, jellifies me longer.

A sudden shock, a noise, getting too cold, a quick, unexpected movement, will also trigger an instant internal reaction. This feels traumatic, brutal, cruel. It feels like dominoes falling internally, click, click, click and with them, as they fall, goes me, endlessly falling off a cliff deeper into a vast chasm of emptiness inside myself.

Not only am I free-falling into oblivion, my mind is falling with me, shutting down, blanking out, fuzzing over, locking me in, one domino at a time, into a tiny space where my thoughts don't work and my words can't get to my mouth in one piece or even materialise in my head. My language, if any is left, is limited, misspoken, coming from a place of deterioration and assault. I cannot literally see clearly. I burn up or freeze with cold, as if icicles hang from my nose. I shake at the beginning and at the end of each bout. Pain already burning me, intensifies and clamours all over my body, louder and louder. My head hurts increasingly. My body numbs. I feel lost in empty pain-filled muscles. My skin crawls with screaming sensations. I feel as if my life, my expectation, my intention and my hope have all been stolen instantly from me, wrecked my tiniest of abilities, battered my senses, consigned me to non-existent being, where nothing is possible, not even thought.

Nothing is tolerated, not even kind words or affectionate, warm, supportive, gentle touch. Nothing is possible, not eating, not drinking, not speaking, not movement. I am stuck where I was for hours literally in agony, stiff on the outside, molten jelly on the inside. I wait. If I feel cross it doesn't help. If I feel hopeful, it doesn't make a difference. If I try to move, it doesn't work. If I want to think about something, I cannot. If I want to scratch an itch, it is not possible. If I am sitting up, unsupported, the most I can do is fall over. If I am lying down, the paralysis is total. My eyes shut and cannot open again. I cannot see. If there is pressure on my head it is extreme pain. Lying still for hours unable to move a millimetre is way beyond uncomfortable. Coming out of paralysis only increases noise, light, movement sensitivity. I am in torment. I cannot access the help I need. I cannot ask for it but I cannot tolerate it either.

> How does this feel to be here again? Beyond words. Beyond understanding. Beyond believable, that this is my life again and again, stuck in intense

agony, unable even to open my lips or move my painfully stuck jaw or toes.

Heels burn in agony. Neck throbs with stiffness. Eyes bulge with itching, burning, throbbing numbness. Stomach, massively swollen presses on my diaphragm, making breathing harder. Bladder presses as paralysis releases me slowly, partially, groggily, painfully back to limited movement and even worse hypersensitivity from every noise, light, movement, smell. Eventually I will be unbound, yet weakened, blanked, emptied of possibility, still in its grips, internally cut off.

How many times have I been paralysed, in the 27 years that I have been severely disabled? How many days, weeks, years, decades lost in repeated paralysis? How many interactions and precious moments have I been robbed of?

Honestly it is a burning, blanked out blur now. I cannot even begin to count them, but a ball park figure of every night's sleep paralysis, alone, is 9,855 times. If I had been paralysed once every day as well as every night, that would have been 19,710 paralyses. But I can be paralysed up to 5 times a day or once all day. It can be total, partial, one-sided, muscles, hands and feet, arms, legs, stomach, throat, mouth, lips, eyes, facial muscles, jaw in any combination, mostly 3/4 of me at least or total is the norm. As paralysis strikes, heart rate shifts, blood pressure is impacted, oxygen SATs can temporarily lower, particularly when lying down.

When I endured building noise that lasted over a period of several years I was paralysed roughly 180 times a month, without adding the sleep paralysis. That is 2,160 times in a single year. Add the sleep paralysis on top and that increases to 2,525 times in those years. If you take an average of 2 extra paralyses a day, it would make a total of 29, 565 paralyses over 27 years. In truth its probably a lot higher than that. In between, there are hours and days of extreme weakness so intense movement is still too difficult. This only includes the most extreme noticeable paralyses.

Whether I am paralysed 5 times a day plus sleep or paralysed once badly all day long, each paralysis equally destroys my life. But sleep paralysis is a little less brutal and somehow less traumatic than the other types I experience.

> Just think about that. An excess of twenty-nine thousand paralyses in twenty-seven years. Paralysis, not just a lack of movement, but affecting me on every level, affecting me internally as well as externally, cognitively as well as physically, blocking both action and interaction.

And then ask, how can it be possible that physical paralysis, recognised by the pioneers as part of the neurological disease, Myalgic Encephalomyelitis, is simply not even acknowledged as a symptom, any more, in the diagnostic criteria they use to identify it?

How on earth can you square that with people like me, diagnosed with Very Severe ME, whose whole lives are dominated by it?

The issue is that ME services should be appropriate to the need, yet fail people experiencing paralysis. Also there is such an apparent lack of understanding as to how easily people can deteriorate massively and then no idea how to help them get back what was lost.

You can, with huge effort, explore paralysis outside of ME, for a comorbid condition or a misdiagnosis, but it still doesn't clarify whether it is part of ME, if it is ignored as a fundamental symptom of ME.

How can we be left in that no man's land for so long, trying to find out what has gone so very wrong and still have no categorical answers or adequate recognition of it?

It is beyond shocking.

> Paralysis in ME has neither been researched nor referred to adequately in literature re ME and is overlooked by most medics who either come across accounts of it from patients or see it first hand. So much to be done to acknowledge this awful physiological occurrence in ME especially to those with Severe ME.
>
> Moira Dillon, ME Advocates Ireland (MEAI)

32

HELPLESS TO GET HELP

∿

Every single moment of paralysis is a moment of indescribable torment and confusion and intolerable pain and indescribable sensations, that rage freely around and inside you, through your skin, your brain, your veins, your muscles, your bones, your blood, your cells, everywhere, on every level, leaving you collapsing and helpless to function.

- You are helpless to get the help you need.
- You are helpless to explain how to help you.
- You are helpless to comprehend communication that might help you.
- You are helpless to be given help and helpless to understand that the person trying to help you is not being clumsy or careless or not trying hard enough, but that you simply cannot bear anyone near you

and you cannot see clearly and even if they were the quietest, most gently, loving, kind, considerate, aware person in the whole world, they would still be hurting you because your body is so unbelievably, implausibly, unimaginably, massively, inexplicably hypersensitive and violated by every normal thing, interaction, presence, person, even kindness to you.

INTRODUCTION TO THE SHEER HELPLESSNESS OF PARALYSIS, BY CHRISTINE FENTON

What follows is an excellent, though painful, description of what people diagnosed with Severe and Very Severe ME, who experience total body paralysis, may go through.

Christine Fenton has suffered long term with this disease and is a passionate ME advocate.

It is important to note that there is little recorded in the history of Myalgic Encephalomyelitis concerning the nature and underlying physiology that results in paralysis, despite it being recognised as a major symptom by the early pioneers.

34

THE SHEER ABSOLUTE HELPLESSNESS OF PARALYSIS, BY CHRISTINE FENTON

~

When I first read Greg's earlier books on Severe ME, I finally found that others experienced paralysis.

Mine is always triggered by an event, that is after seriously going beyond my boundaries.

I cannot open my eyes, move, speak but can hear, everything is sensitised, pain increases, my body will jump off the bed involuntarily at the sound of someone putting a cup onto a saucer but I cannot create movement.

My dentist has witnessed it and calls it a neurological shut down.

My extremities go cold, heart rate slows and BP drops. My core is hot and will cause concern as the temperature reaches 37.6, but no one feels the freezing limbs.

I can think, but cannot create speech. I 'speak' to myself in my head about what the nurses/ED staff don't understand as they do the opposite of what I need, shouting at me, *'Christine, Christine, can you hear me, open your eyes if you can hear me.'* I can hear them, they're hurting me by shouting and touching the bed but I can't respond.

'She's in a coma, her eyes are flicking' (as I try with my soul to open my eyes but only the lashes flicker as the single result for the immense effort) and I hear the proclamation *'she's having an epileptic fit'*. No, I'm just trying to open my eyes.

The sheer absolute helplessness of knowing that this will pass, but unknowing healthcare staff and Doctors will, unknowingly, inflict more pain and discomfort on my tortured body before, finally, I am able to communicate my needs.

It takes about four hours before I can create speech, actual spoken words. I think them, plan them, then when I have the energy to push a whispered word from my mouth, a beyond endurance effort to reach out and explain my need, it's not heard or is dismissed.

If, a massive if, someone will take my hand and ask me a question requiring a *'Yes'* answer, *'Christine can you hear me?'* quietly and close to my ear, and if they give me time to get my brain to send a message to my finger, a brain which has shut down the pathways which create movement and if I use an immense effort to create a signal to move I can respond by a slight finger tip movement, but the person asking the question needs to be sensitive to the slightest fingertip movement as that's all I have and it drains me.

The energy used to create that whisper of communication has exhausted me and I have to wait to recover in order to try again, to try to communicate the paralysis to an unhearing hospital.

It's taken me several years to have a Care Plan in place which describes the paralysis so that now I'm put on appropriate treatment, so I rest and the energy which is focused solely on the essential organs is not further drained by the environment around me.

Sometimes the paralysis only affects my limbs and I can speak, slowly to explain my needs, but I still need to explain why I need the specific treatment that will aid my recovery; they don't understand.

It has taken years of torture to arrive at a situation where my needs are on paper and those who know me in the hospital are aware and prepared.

If I meet staff new to me, who haven't read the Care Plan, as they know best, then I will enter the same living hell.

I'm lucky, hell passes.

It takes weeks to recover from the onslaught, maybe months to regain an earlier baseline, if I do and I do reach a higher level of function which makes me one of the lucky people with ME, as I can engage in life in those better times.

Dare I think of a time when hell doesn't pass? No, I don't think I'm strong enough to contemplate such a state and I am strong, incredibly so, but living in that horrendous, less than life state, is a situation beyond my contemplation.

My love and thoughts to Linda and those who experience very severe ME & to those, like Greg, who care with love; the source of the strength to enable the soul to survive.

35
CONTEMPLATE PARALYSIS IF YOU CAN

∽

Stop what you are doing, right this moment.
That means you cannot move any part of you.
Your feet are stuck to the ground.
Your thighs and your bottom are stuck to the seat, whatever your position was, when it hit you.
You cannot change to a more comfortable position, not even an inch.
Your toes are immobile, your hands are useless, your fingers too will not move a fraction.
You have an itch on your face, another coming to your head.
But, you cannot move to scratch them.
They are irritating, but impossible to reach.
So however itchy or demanding the itches become, you still cannot move to scratch them.
Of course you want to. It is a simple enough gesture, quick

as a flash in the normal moving world. But no, you cannot move your finger, lift your arm, find your face, move your head, even a degree from where it currently is.

None of these movements are possible, all removed from possibility in one bizarre instant, beyond your control.

Now your heals are really hurting from the pressure on them.

Your calf muscles are beginning to burn with a hotter sensation of pain, but inside that, they are feeling weird and weak, empty.

No strength.

Nothing.

Numbness is spreading deeper and wider over your whole body.

Your back muscles are beginning to go into spasm.

The pain is starting to scream at you, as your muscles feel like they are crashing and dissolving, breaking down from solid to fragmented strings and fractured cells.

You need to move.

You need to lie down, but your head is hurting and there is nothing you can do to help yourself, except stay calm and try to think.

Thinking though is becoming harder.

You feel as if you have been pushed away from the outside world, like you are disappearing inside a deep inner chasm.

You are losing your ability to focus.

Your eyes are staring.

Your sight is kind of darkened and patchy.

You feel like you are dissolving into nothing.

Your thoughts are harder to find.

You want to talk, you want to say something, but by now

your mouth is stuck shut, your lips feel zipped together, your jaw is clenched tight.

You cannot speak a word.

You know what you want to say.

There are so many things you need and want to say right now, but the thoughts, are now disappearing from view.

The pathway to speak has been mysteriously withdrawn.

You cannot ask for the drink you need.

You cannot say you need food, medicine, a blanket or any of the things that might help you.

If you are alone, you cannot call for help.

If you are not alone, you cannot tell the person what you want.

You might manage a grunt or some prearranged sound, but even this may be too much.

No energy to breathe?

No strength in the muscles?

The pain is sneaking more intensely up your body.

Your diaphragm is struggling.

Your chest muscles are burning with pain.

Your face is hurting.

Your eyes are throbbing and dry and may have shut and now refuse to open, despite all commands you can internally send them.

You are really struggling, now.

If you are lucky you may be able to fall to the side and lie down.

You may break out of it for a moment at best and move a limb or tip yourself sideways.

Or your body may just give way so you fall over.

But that is it.

Your breathing, shallow, sounds and feels as if you have gone to sleep.

But you haven't!

You are still conscious and awake inside your mind.

But nothing is working.

Everything hurts.

Everything is impossible and your bladder is getting desperate now.

But no, you cannot bear to be touched or moved.

Even if you have a wheelchair, you cannot tolerate movement.

You cannot bear being lifted.

You cannot bear motion or movement.

You cannot sit upright.

You cannot be helped in that moment, no matter how great the need.

You cannot go to the toilet, even though you are desperate.

There is no strength in you.

Your muscles will not comply, cannot hold you up, cannot perform the simplest task to help yourself.

Your tongue is numb.

Your lips are numb.

You cannot lick them or open them to speak and say what you need.

This is the place you repeatedly return to, with potentially multiple triggers of paralysis.

This is the invisible, empty, darkened place you inhabit, waiting for the shift to come once more and movement gradually to come back to you, ever so slowly and gradually.

It never leaves.

It always lurks.

Weakness dominates internally.

Numbness and pain define your boundary or disappear your edges, so that proprioception is lost.

Your face may feel as if it has no definition at all.

Your muscles may tremor or shake going in or coming out of paralysis.

The spasms can be strong, violent, repeated, uncontrollable.

This is your life.

This is your body, though it no longer responds to you and you feel trapped inside it, floating in suspended animation.

Hours, day, weeks, decades go by and you are still following the same rhythm that paralysis sets out for you.

One minute you may be able to move, one minute it may be gone.

One moment you may suddenly have lost your hand or arm, your fingers, your feet, your whole left side or your mouth, your eyes or literally everything.

That is the horror of periodic, repeat paralysis, never knowing when it will come, but never quite leaving you either......

Stop what you are doing right now and be prepared to lose all possibility, all plans, all intention, all the things you take for granted.

It is hard to imagine or be able to stay that still, unless you have this.

But if you just stop and reflect upon it, for even a few minutes, you might start to become aware of how shattering it might be to experience it, to imagine all the things you would have lost out on, all the dashed hopes, all the lost connections and activities, how uncomfortable, painful, agonising, it must be, how dependent it would make you on others, how inaccessible the simplest thing you take for granted would be, like scratching your head or reading a book, making a drink, answering the phone, speaking to anyone, getting something to eat, even sitting upright.

And what is worse, it is utterly beyond your control.

For this is an absolutely life changing reality!

And it never goes away.

36

BRAIN FOG IN SEVERE AND VERY SEVERE ME

"**B**RAIN FOG" IS SUCH AN inadequate term to describe the devastating, sometimes profound level of Cognitive Dysfunction that people may suffer, in Severe/Very Severe ME.

Cognitive Dysfunction is a major, grossly misunderstood symptom.

People are likely to have MASSIVE problems with:

- Receiving information.
- Processing information.
- Comprehending the content of conversation.
- Remembering names of people.
- Remembering the names of common things.
- Forgetting information.
- Forgetting what they are saying mid-sentence.

- Not being able to articulate or speak the thought they have in their head.
- Having a completely blank mind.
- Loss of internal visual imagery.
- Spelling difficulties.
- Mathematical difficulties.
- Poor short-term memory.
- A disconnection between thought and action and thought and vision.
- Using the completely wrong word even though the person knows what they want to say.
- Getting distracted by other thoughts and saying the wrong thing.
- External noise disturbing the ability to think.
- Unable to understand or take in information if there is another noise in the room.
- Saying words in the wrong order, back to front or swapping first letters of consecutive words.
- Forgetting what they are doing.
- Task confusion, for example putting something in completely the wrong place.
- Not being able to think about or express the thing they need to think about.
- Difficulties coordinating thought, word and action.
- Difficulties with exchange of information.
- Difficulty with processing and answering questions.
- Difficulty following fast speech.
- Difficulty tolerating loud speech.
- Difficulty understanding the meaning of information.
- Difficulty following instructions.

- Difficulty understanding descriptive information leading to mental overload.

If a person says they cannot do something, even talk or listen to you or understand what you are saying or bear your presence near them or in the room at all, then it is absolutely essential to respect and accept or try to understand this; not ignore it or think that you know better.

Try again later. Please NEVER neglect the person because things are difficult, but always respect their reality even if you cannot fully comprehend it.

For the person who cannot comprehend or process what you are saying it can be very difficult. This is also true for the person trying to communicate with them. Great compassion, patience and integrity are needed, to wait for a better moment to interact or to find an alternative way to communicate.

CAN YOU POSSIBLY IMAGINE WHAT THAT IS LIKE? No, you can't.

Can you develop empathy? Hopefully.

37

HOW TO SUPPORT SOMEONE WITH SLEEP DYSFUNCTION

~

THE PERSON MAY BE AWAKE at night, disturbed, uncomfortable, in need of assistance, unable to get to sleep or gain rest. Their normal sleep pattern may be grossly disrupted. They may get little or no restorative sleep. They may experience real problems going off to sleep and/or difficulties in waking.

- They may experience insomnia at night and sleep all day.
- They may wake frequently, due to pain, need to urinate, discomfort, needing help to turn or something else.
- Their minds may be overloaded and racing.
- They may sleep more than normal.
- Body functions may be altered, ie may need to urinate more frequently at night.

- Thirst or hunger may be increased.
- They may need particular medicine at set times or for a specific issue.
- Their body-clock may be out of sync.
- Blood sugar may be low.
- They may have vivid dreams.
- They may choose to stay up later or get up during the night if they are wide awake.

Care Skills and Knowledge

These are some possible skills that might be required. Everyone is different. This is not a full list. The more severely ill person may need very specific highly trained skills to meet their particular individual needs which may not be covered here.

Never do anything without agreement from the person. Always flow with the person. Know what you need to know to enable basic needs to be met: toilet, food, drinks, medicine, comfort etc. The person may need frequent physical and/or emotional help and support throughout the night.

- Know how to assist someone in bed.
- Know how to give a bed bath, if it will help the person.
- Know how to work safely in low light.
- Know how to help someone drink through a straw.
- Learn any lifting techniques taught.
- Be trained in how to safely use of a hoist.
- Develop skills in how to safely manoeuvre a sensitive, weakened person in a wheelchair, possibly through doorways and along narrow corridors.
- Aquire knowledge of dietary need.

- Aquire knowledge of how to aid transfer to a toilet and back to a wheelchair.
- Learn to work with other professionals involved.
- Be aware of specific sensitivities and how to care in those circumstances, for example, noise sensitivity, light sensitivity, motion and movement sensitivity, touch sensitivity.
- Learn how to be flexible and adapt to the need, which may vary.
- Get used to helping at odd hours.
- Do not judge the person or blame them, rather be encouraging and supportive.

38

PAIN IN VERY SEVERE ME

∼

IN THE MOST SEVERE forms of ME, pain may feel like being assaulted physically inside and outside in multiple ways, all at the same time, with no relief or escape. It may feel like having the blankest emptiest space in your head where everything beautiful, colourful, creative, every image, every comprehension, every hope, dream, expectation and every possibility is extinguished, except for the blank swirling pressure and piercing pain that hurts you.

It may feel like having a knife twisted into the centre of your head whilst at the same time clashing pots and pans as loud as possible in your ears, so that it jangles round your head for hours and hours and hours, after every single noise has gone away, whilst having a massive heavy, hammer repeatedly hit against your head continuously, so that you cannot think and you cannot escape and you cannot stop it and you cannot bear it, but you have to endure it, with no alleviation or protection from it and no prediction of when it will increase and no knowledge of whether it will stop, going on seemingly endlessly.

> You may not be able to explain, to articulate, to comprehend, to convey, to speak, to describe, to identify the horror of your reality inside and out; the clashing, clanging crashing reality of central nervous system dysfunction causing utterly destructive mayhem in your head and body.

It may feel like burning with pain on the inside, so that even your bones feel on fire and your skin is screaming at you, as crawling, irritating, nothingness reverberates around your body and all over your itching, burning skin, so that every contact feels like it will crush you and the pressure of contact is so unbearable that you want to scream forever with the pain of it and the indescribable nature of it, where even the air around you hurts to be invaded and feels as if you have been banged into, even if there is no physical contact at all.

> Your head might be so intensely agonised that you think you will surely die from the extreme indescribable throbbing, burning, piercing, vastness of agony. Even though you feel you cannot survive or bear any physical contact, yet still you want someone to come and take the pain away, but there is no one to help you and there is nothing to alleviate it and it goes on and on and on and on for hours and days and weeks and even months, year

in, year out, yet every second feels like it will surely be your last, because there is no pain greater, possible.

INTRODUCTION TO "PAIN" POEM BY EMILY COLLINGRIDGE

Often paralysed and tube fed, Emily Collingridge, in this poem published on Stonebird, described the unimaginable pain she was in; pain only relieved by high dose morphine. She was treated with drugs normally reserved for patients undergoing chemotherapy, her nausea was so extreme. She could not bear light, sound, touch or movement. In 2010 Emily published "Severe ME/CFS : A Guide to Living", written during a short period of respite from her most extreme symptoms, the first comprehensive reference book to exist on Severe ME. Emily died, in hospital, in 2012.

40

PAIN, BY EMILY COLLINGRIDGE

∼

I am being beaten, my side kicked, my face stamped on.
It's crushed and caving in on itself, the cheek feels thick
    and swollen
I must look hideously deformed
Now my insides are being hollowed out and replaced
    with an acid
The weight of the liquid makes my limbs heavy and pins
    me to the bed
The acid burns everything it touches so I am being worn
    away from the inside out
I try to lie still, but this does not stop it from sloshing
    back and forth
Back and forth, back and forth
Spreading from the left hand side across my shoulders
    to the limbs on the right
Something cold and sharp is piercing my skull

It makes my stomach heave
There's no way of getting remotely comfortable now
Pain is screaming from so many different parts of
 my body
I don't know which to listen to
The noise is deafening
It's driving me insane and taking my breath away
Surely this is the point in the nightmare when I must sit
 upright in one sudden movement
Gasp for breath
And then feel everything recede
But no, it does not happen
I am not asleep
So on the screaming inside me goes
Relentless
Somehow sleep does come
But the pain manages to follow me in and take over my
 dreams
More screaming
Now it releases itself from my throat in small moans

My mother tries to comfort me
But even when I stir and wake I do not hear her
I have lost the boundary that defines reality
I have been consumed by pain
Pain is the only reality
I want a way out
Any way out
Oblivion
Peace
All those drug related words, that's what I seek
I do not truly want my life to be over

But I am alone in fighting this
And the pain feels stronger than I am

I am lost, worn out and weepy
What now?
I rest, I wait, I blot out the screaming.

INTRODUCTION TO MY COPING MECHANISM BY CORINA DUYN

Corina Duyn is a powerful advocate for people with ME in Ireland.

She also is an amazing and talented poet and artist, who loves to create puppets, art and books to express her experience, as well as enabling others to express themselves, too.

She finds that beauty, nature and creativity have helped her to cope with the many physically isolated years of living with Severe ME.

It was my joy and honour to be the first student on her online Puppet Making Course. From a distance Corina taught me how to make "Johnny Toes", my very own puppet - I was so delighted that I wrote a song about the experience and posted it on YouTube:[1]

A true teacher has to be innovative, imaginative and flexible, that was certainly my experience with Corina. For me, an isolated home-carer, Corina's course helped me to focus upon and affirm my own creativity, that is so important!

It is creativity, the wonder of the garden and nature that help Corina cope with the pain and the isolation of her ever-changing illness, as she explains in this beautiful piece.

Like her, they too, nurture my soul.

---

1. "Here Comes Johnny Toes!" https://www.youtube.com/watch?v=WQhZYDeS1pk

42

MY COPING MECHANISM BY CORINA DUYN

∼

ILLNESS LIKE M.E. is certainly not a linear experience. I have (too many) days I am so totally exhausted, unwell and in a lot of pain. Yet, my creative mind even then comes up with thoughts on how to depict this through imagery. This, I believe is part of my coping mechanism to stay afloat. Imagery and words help me to figure out the reality of this every challenge and changing illness. At times it is just all too much. Even my beautiful home and garden feels too much. And at the same time my home and garden envelop me with such beauty and gratitude that I can not imagine being in a different physical space.

Yesterday I rested in the garden, and also explored the beautiful poppies again. What they tell me is that there is 'beauty in decay'. It is important to keep looking at what is beautiful and good and stunning and wonderful. Life is not only good when all is as we wish it to be.

Look at the stunning poppy, in transition from perfect flower to stunning seed head - All the seed full of promise of a new life.

All these moments of life nurture my soul, just like my creative mind.

USEFUL SYMPTOM EXPERIENCE RECORD CHART

∼

It may help to keep a record of symptoms to compare over time or record important information and any changes. We use this basic one. This is only an example. You may want to make your own, based on your own symptom experience and need.

HEALTH CHART

- Bed time previous night
- Wake time(s)
- Up time
- Ph urine
- Oxygen level
- Heart rate
- Breakfast

- Snack
- Lunch
- Snack
- Dinner
- Drinks
- Paralysed from sleep
- No of times paralysed in the day
- Length of times paralysed
- Posture paralysed
- Other triggers of paralysis
- Headache
- Length of duration of headache
- Head pain
- Eye pain
- Pins and Needles
- Numbness
- Nausea/vomiting
- Upset tummy
- Swollen tummy
- Sweating/temperature variability
- Pain level
- Mood
- Mind
- Spasms
- Energy
- Allergy
- Extra issues
- Bed time tonight
- Drugs

44

INTRODUCTION TO CAN A CARE PLAN HELP TO ENSURE I HAVE A 'POSITIVE EXPERIENCE OF CARE'? BY CHRISTINE FENTON

I have great pleasure in sharing Christine Fenton's informative and moving piece on the need for a Care Plan. Based on her experience in Eire it outlines areas that may be incorporated into a Care Plan in order to try and get care needs safely met in Hospital.

45

CAN A CARE PLAN HELP TO ENSURE I HAVE A 'POSITIVE EXPERIENCE OF CARE'? BY CHRISTINE FENTON

∼

MY EXPERIENCES OF ACUTE CARE, through many admissions, led me to understand that even if I had a supportive Consultant, and not everyone can find one of those, when my Consultant wasn't available and as an inpatient you don't see them everyday, I was still at the mercy of 'the view of ME' held by every other member of staff I met, Doctors, Nurses, Occupational Therapists, Physiotherapists etc. and their associated view of me: a person who just needed to pull herself together and make an effort, after all there was nothing physically wrong as evidenced by 'normal blood' tests and everyone gets tired, any parent, carer or those working long hours can attest to understanding 'chronic fatigue' and they can push through so why don't I?

My voice counted for nothing. Trying to explain my needs, what ME is and how it affects me when at my weakest or exacerbated my symptoms, I achieved nothing, as no one was willing to listen. When paralysed I couldn't communicate, so suffered until eventually I could try to get the attention of a member of staff. Quite simply I suffered so many indignities and inappropriate care during admissions that returning to a pre-admission baseline took months if it was achieved at all.

I had to find a way to prevent the harm caused by being admitted.

I decided that putting the things I needed, but was too unwell to communicate onto paper, would help. I created an Emergency File which went everywhere with me. My Consultant agreed and was willing to provide input and subsequently sign the sheets I created. Even with this, no one else accepted them, they had no currency in hospital services.

The sheets described how my body experienced different parts of the hospital and how best to provide appropriate supports.

For instance, if taken into the Emergency Department, telling me to 'take a seat' was a totally inappropriate request, which did not take into account my needs. Sitting upright is guaranteed to make me deteriorate, the worse I am to start with, the faster that deterioration is.

One memorable time, after being at an Out Patients Appointment and becoming unwell, the Clinic staff were able to find a Porter but no trolley, so my Personal Assistant (yes, I'm lucky enough to have a Care Package to enable me to live at home) scooted 'the body' on my mobility scooter round to the Emergency Department. She explained that I needed to be flat, NOW, and passed over the relevant sheet from the Emergency File, which explained my needs, signed by my Consultant.

The Receptionist had no idea what to do. My body gave up

and I slid to the floor, as a graceful slide beats hitting it with a thump!!

A Nurse came over and said 'you can't lie there this is a busy department!'

Given the choice would I want to lie on the floor?! A Porter arrived, with a trolley and a hoist was obtained to lift 'the body' onto the trolley. I could speak but had by this time lost the use of my arms and legs, a partial paralysis which is too common an experience when my body has exceeded its limits. I was not triaged, no medical observations such as BP, heart rate etc were done and I was shoved up against a wall in the corridor.

Fortunately, shortly after, my Consultant happened to be passing and intervened, so I was whizzed into a cubicle and the plan we had in place for my care was followed.

Had he not been passing, I would have been left in a corridor to deteriorate, despite having a PA with me, as the power of the hospital is stronger than the voice of those visiting it.

Subsequently, after my supportive Consultant left the hospital I submitted a complaint, which referenced the standard of care the health service said every patient should expect and the fact that I was not receiving that care.

I need to be clear that I had made a number of complaints in the past but these were minimised and nothing changed so I had, over years, ensured that every time 'something' happened in hospital, I wrote my version of the incident and sent that in, asking for it to be included in my medical records. In this way, the somewhat biased narrative of healthcare professionals with a very judgmental view of ME and me, which was recorded in the records, a narrative which hinted at me not coping, being anxious, there being a psychological component etc, was balanced by my experience, the Patient's voice and where I could find relevant research then links to documents which anchored my perspective in medical research. Doctors are big on 'evidence-based medicine' so I sought to provide them with the evidence they have not time to find or read or maybe they don't choose to?

Over a period of time I recorded patterns of behaviour in the hospital, by Doctors and Nurses which identified a less than appropriate standard of care.

Having said that, I also experienced staff who are vocationally gifted and always did their best for me.

I had met similar problems in dealing with the local Disability Services. Their judgements, based on a total ignorance of ME, were written into the record with a clear intent to label me as 'not coping' and being unreasonable in my expectations. What is in those records hurts to this day, those wounds have never healed. When I first read my records I was astounded that any professional could mis-represent an individual in such a way and that they could remove the Patient's voice from the record was beyond my comprehension.

Again, I began to ensure my voice was added to the record, by writing my record of the Patient perspective of every interaction and emailing it so my voice could not be 'disappeared' from the record.

Adding my voice to my medical records was the best thing I could have done as prior to that the records contained only a health service narrative, which evidenced limited, if any, knowledge of ME and a non-evidence based judgement that the problem was psychological.

I then submitted a complaint which was investigated independently of the health service. The complaint was upheld and returned thirty-three recommendations which related to the hospital and to the local disability services as well as some for the whole health service as well.

Of greatest benefit was that the Investigators saw the benefits of the Emergency File and recommended that, until there was clinical guidance on ME for the country, the Emergency File should be followed.

In 2019 I was facing the first admission since the Investigation and it was agreed that the Emergency File should become a formalised personal Care Plan, which was accepted by the hospital and which had to be followed.

The only thing was, I had to write it, as there was no knowledge in the hospital (or the health service) which enabled them to do so!

It would have been lovely to have a collaborative approach, but that just isn't available between health services and people with ME, as we hold the knowledge of the biomedical presentation and other than a few individuals, acute medical professionals do not.

My approach was based upon two themes:

1) Providing accessible learning for health professionals about ME.

2) What 'My Needs' are, based on the experience of several admissions, for each aspect of acute care.

I decided it was important to include the medical classifications which Patients don't usually have to memorise, but for those with ME, reminding Consultants that ME is classified as a neurological disorder using their own language, is a gentle nudge in the right direction.

USEFUL CLASSIFICATIONS:
WHO ICD 10 G93.3 Neurological Disorder

SNOMED SCTID: 118940003 Disorder of the nervous system (Disorder)

I also decided to remind staff of the quality standards of the health service I was using. Every health-service has a Charter or some document, which informs Patients of the standard of care they should expect to receive.

A Patient is entitled to be informed of the benefits, risks and alternatives to any proposed treatment.

There is a right to consent.

There is a right to dignity and respect.

For a Health Service to fulfil the above commitments *'My Needs'* have to be a part of the conversation and may not be ignored.

If they are, please make your voice heard by putting in a complaint as the likelihood is you will be heard more clearly!

∽

My Care Plan includes my presentation and needs in each part of the acute journey.

(a generic example is available on MEAI blogspot.

1. **Contact Details**

Next of Kin/Carer/PA/GP/Pharmacy/Consultant etc.

2. **Diagnoses**

All your relevant diagnoses.

3. **Do/Do Not and Patient's Vital Signs**

Make clear what harms you or causes deterioration

If you have low BP/subnormal temperature etc record it, as hospitals assess people against 'standard' measures, which may result in a Dr missing something important when assessing you.

4. **Ambulance**

What do ambulance staff need to know about you?
What are your needs?
Cover your eyes/ears?
Keep you warm or cool?

5. EMERGENCY DEPARTMENT (ED)

You may go to ED by car or by ambulance.

If you arrive by car you will be asked to wait until a Nurse sees you to do an initial assessment. Then, if not classed as an emergency, you will be asked to wait.

What are your needs?

Is there anything in the waiting area which affects you, being upright, lights, aromas etc?

If there is inform the staff immediately.

Make sure you take sufficient food/liquids and meds to enable you to survive an ED wait!

6. AT MY WORST I AM ....

Describe what you experience when you are at your worst, when you deteriorate, what is your experience of yourself, which is a pattern you've experienced several times.

This lets the Doctors know this is not a one-off event but part of a pattern of deterioration which needs to be pro-actively managed.

7. INPATIENT INFORMATION:

What do staff need to know to enable you to pace?

If you're admitted to a ward, the standard practice in a hospital is to get Patients mobilised. It is really hard for a person with ME to override the drive to get you to be active, be out of bed, follow the ward routine.

Ensure you describe what happens when you exceed your energy limits.

Explain that being pushed to go beyond your known limits <u>**increases the risk of you being harmed**</u>, that is you will deteriorate and describe how that deterioration is experienced; being unable to sit up, unable to eat etc.

One really important point for me was that staff were to ensure the call bell was placed IN my hand. Too many times I have been paralysed and the call bell has been lying on the bed, a million miles away. In my hand, with sheer will and effort, I can press it and call for help.

Describe the things you need to manage YOUR energy.

If a hospital has been warned of a risk and ignores it, you are in a good position to hold them to account.

Hospital's do not like the word risk!

If you need help to eat or to wash or need activities spread across the day, describe that.

If nursing staff appear not to hear you, I suggest asking to speak with the Ward Sister and if there's no joy there, ask to speak with a nursing supervisor.

8. Surgery and Dental Treatment:

Important considerations

There are materials in the ME world which describe the risks associated with such interventions and how best to minimise deterioration, by avoiding certain drugs commonly used in anaesthetics for instance.

Do your research and put the information and the link to your source in writing.

9. Discharge Planning:

Preparing for discharge and identifying supports needed

You 'should' be involved in planning your discharge.

Be very clear that you communicate your needs.

If reliant on care at home, have your care needs increased?

How will these be met?

Can you travel home by car?

Do you need an ambulance?

Can you go home or do you need to consider a nursing home for a while to help you improve?

Do you need nutritional foods on prescription?

If you have reached the point where you need support to be able to live at home, make sure that this is fully discussed and an assessment for community supports is done BEFORE you are discharged.

10. OUTPATIENT ATTENDANCE:

What are your needs at an Out-Patients appointment?

Short waiting times, a quiet or dim area, wheelchair accessible, a place you can put your legs up or recline/lie down etc.

Be Aware: Having your Consultant's or GPs support for your Care Plan is important, but it will still likely be ignored by other health professionals. Putting your needs on paper is an empowering act as Your Voice, on paper, in your medical records makes it much harder for staff to ignore you as paper is a tool which aids accountability!

If those living with ME have to hold our health services to account by teaching them how to care for us, then so be it, we're a capable bunch and we can hold our health services to account by telling them what we need them to know.

NEXT ADMISSION

Once the hospital agreed to the Care Plan, the next admission, which included a General Anaesthetic and a minor procedure, resulted in a three week stay and a couple of step backs, resulting in paralysis, but the Care Plan made the experience hundreds of time better than ever before, the best I have ever had. Every member of staff was aware and supportive, the difference was incredible, I felt safe.

I cannot stress the importance of telling the hospital of your needs in advance and requiring them to care for you with dignity and respect.

We shouldn't have to explain our illness, we should be being guided and supported, but for the moment, we are required to guide the healthcare professionals who engage with us, so take on the role of an equal partner in your care, respect their medical experience and expect them to respect your experience of your body in a collaborative partnership in which you work together to discover the best ways to manage your care.

It took me nine years to achieve what should be the basics of care, I hope your journey is a shorter one.

PART THREE: ON THE CARING ROLE

Here we take a look at what it means and what it takes to care, in the face of profound illness, complex disability, multiple hypersensitivities, paralysis, agony, cognitive dysfunction and multi-system dysfunction.

Time and time again we will come back to the most important issue and that is you and your values, your attitude, your posture, your commitment, your awareness and your openness to learning; for upon these all else depends.

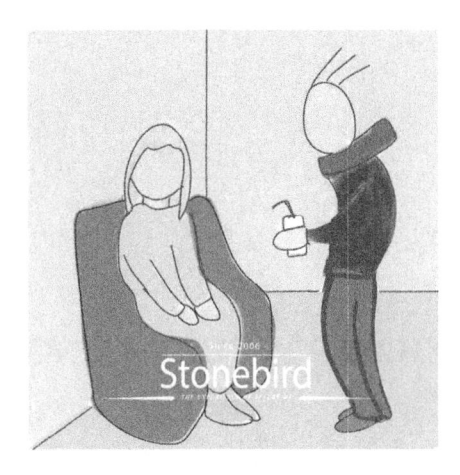

Even if you cannot move, even if you cannot communicate, even if you cannot think, still you are precious and your presence matters.

47

VAST CHASM

∼

This is a poem raising awareness of the huge difference between you and the person you are trying to help. [1]It is so important to try and begin to comprehend that there is a vast chasm between your experience and theirs.

>For the person who can do things,
>Easily simply quickly,
>Who can comprehend conversation just like that,
>Who can read and comprehend instantly,
>Who can think about something and speak it
>Or think about something and write it
>Or think about something and tell someone else
>By phone, by letter, by email, by speech
>Or think about something and then take action,
>It is impossibly hard to begin to comprehend
>The interior world of the Very Severe ME sufferer,

Where there are blocks
And breaks
And disjointedness,
Where simplicity and flow should be
And where fog bathes everything in impossible
Lack of clarity,
Where inner vision is lost,
Where thoughts do not hold together
Into a coherent view,
Where memory
Dissolves
And words will not materialise,
Where even if you have an idea inside your head
There is no pathway to the outside,
Where the pathways from your brain
To your hand or foot
No longer exists,
Where life in all its fullness
And richness
Is simply missing,
Where forward thought and planning
Are impossible
And even continuity and fluidity of moments
Are broken,
Jagged,
Lost
In the terrible deep emptiness, that resides in ME.
Yet this is the world I exist in
And this is my life
Fractured as it is
By impossibility.
And so this is the world that you too must enter into,

If there is any hope that you will be able
To reach out and help
Not harm me further.

---

1. One British study comparing functioning in people with ME vs people with rheumatoid arthritis, cancer and depression showed a staggering reduction in functioning in ME patients; all the functional health scores were dramatically worse in ME patients. (Nacul et al (2011) **The functional status and well being of people with myalgic encephalomyelitis/chronic fatigue syndrome and their carers** https://bmcpublichealth.biomedcentral.com/articles/10.1186/1471-2458-11-402)

WHO CARES FOR ME? A UNIVERSAL CARE APPROACH TO MYALGIC ENCEPHALOMYELITIS (ME)

O*N STONEBIRD WE STATE ' you don't have to do anything to be of beauty and value in the world. Even if you cannot move, even if you cannot communicate, even if you cannot think, still you are precious and your presence matters'*; that defines our approach to caring.

WHAT IS ME?

Myalgic Encephalomyelitis (ME) is a WHO classified multi-systemic neurological disease. It was originally identified as an enteroviral illnesses.[1] People with Severe and Very Severe ME are so ill that most people cannot easily or safely participate in ordinary life or perform basic living tasks without help. The most severely affected are unable to leave the house, could be confined to bed and spend many hours if not all day, incapacitated and unable to help themselves. They may use wheelchairs part or full- time and are barely able to move.

Their lives are severely isolated. The suffering of the most ill is often invisible and unrecognised.

There is no cure. There is no consistent or universal treatment. The pain of Severe/Very Severe ME is so extreme that drugs may not touch it, many are forced to take extremely strong drugs to gain minimal reductions in pain level. Others have no pain relief at all due to their acute drug sensitivity.

[2]There are a range of serious physical symptoms, with underlying neuro- immune and other physiological implications.

> Currently there is no biomedical pathway in the UK to help recognise, investigate and validate the most severe symptoms and extreme suffering that people endure, often for decades on end, once diagnosed.

A person with ME, with any level of illness, whether mild, moderate or severe can always become more ill, especially if exposed to wrong treatment and inappropriate expectations and demands to do more. It is extremely easy to trigger a deterioration of symptoms.

Never ignore a person's symptoms thinking that they can just push through them.

Why do people need care?

In Very Severe ME, in our experience, the symptoms are present all the time, however they can worsen with exertion, which results in post-exertional deterioration. People either do not have the energy to begin with, to even perform every day tasks, let alone have a quality of life or they run out of energy trying to meet basic needs, then deteriorate and become incapacitated by debilitating, multiple symptoms, such as:

- Pain
- Muscle weakness and muscle fatigue
- Sleep difficulty
- Numbness
- Paralysis
- Muscle spasm
- Cognitive dysfunction
- Noise sensitivity (Hyperacusis)
- Light sensitivity (Photophobia)
- Touch sensitivity (Hyperesthesia)
- Movement sensitivity
- Chemical and perfume sensitivity (Multiple Chemical Sensitivity)
- Gut issues, swallowing difficulty and gastroparesis
- Heart and blood pressure issues
- Dysautonomia

Rest brings temporary, little or no relief, depending on the severity of illness. The suffering and the consequences of over-exertion are often invisible, making it sometimes hard for people to understand why care may be needed.

People with Severe and Very Severe ME need care to survive. They may suffer intensely without relief, yet accessing that care is extremely difficult because of the nature and severity of their symptoms.

Care needs to be provided in an extraordinarily aware and sensitive fashion, understanding that any wrong move, demand or action may lead to unimaginable deterioration and long term consequences.

The ordinary things that people take for granted every day become things that fail to get done and in the worst, most severe forms of ME, they become absolutely intolerable and incredibly difficult to manage, even with help available.

Things like getting dressed, washing your hair, cleaning your teeth, making a phone call, writing a letter, understanding a bill, dealing with problems, filing things away, chatting for even a few minutes to a friend or giving care instructions, all become a complex activity that are literally beyond possible, yet not necessarily explicable as to why they are so hard or not achievable.

Communication is a massively complex issue that people face in getting their needs met and this needs to be understood.

∽

A FLEXIBLE APPROACH TO CARE.

Your presence is of the utmost importance:

1 All you say and do.

2 How you are feeling in yourself.

3 Your energy level.

4 What you are conveying non-verbally towards the other person.

5 Your values and attitudes.

These are all key to interacting well with anyone, but especially so with people who are in high physical pain with a range of tormenting, unremitting, very severe symptoms.

It is important that you know how the slightest wrong movement, noise or action, on your part, may lead to even worsening levels of symptom experience and physical distress. You cannot afford to not be ultra-aware of the potential to do harm.

Every nuance, every breath, every movement counts and can bring relief or negatively impact the person.

A flexible, aware, moment by moment approach is key to successful interaction or at least as a way to try to minimise the risk of triggering deterioration and indescribable additional physical suffering.

To care for someone with Very Severe ME you need to know how to:

Maximise the
Opportunity to
Meet
Each
Need
Tenderly

This says it all. We call it the "MOMENT Approach".

It recognises how each moment is significant and that care may be better provided and interaction may be easier or possible, in some moments more than others.

Remember EVERY moment is a moment when the person is ill. Some moments can feel a lot worse than others.

With Severe and Very Severe ME the suffering and symptoms are continuous; there may be no moment when interaction or meeting care needs is tolerable, due to the intense unrelenting severity of symptoms.

The best moment to approach the person and help them, must be determined in partnership, together, so that you gently help, not inadvertently make things a lot worse for the person.

It is not only that you need to know about the illness and how it impacts the person you help, you need to know specifically, exactly and accurately, what needs doing to help the person and most importantly of all, you specifically need to know the 'how' of caring, which is essential to get right.

This takes:

Respect both of the person as an equal and respect for the illness itself, that ME is a neurological disease, certainly not caused by maladaptive thinking or deconditioning.

Tenderness of approach, as it makes such a difference.

Commitment to learn what is required and to get the care right.

Knowledge about the illness, the unique symptom experience of the person you care for and how you affect the person directly.

Willingness to grow and learn. It requires the highest level of comprehension, plus a willingness to understand that this is not like any other ordinary illness that you will come across.

An ability to change habits that are not appropriate or helpful. You must learn to do things specifically as required by the person, not just the way you may think they should be done. This requires enormous sensitivity, humility and willingness to change.

Awareness that untold harm can occur if you do not notice that things in the environment, especially the impact of your presence for example, how loud you are, whether you remembered not to wear perfume, whether you know that you do not just switch on lights without warning. Each person will have different issues that you will need to be acutely aware of. That awareness must be incorporated into all that you do.

Focus on every aspect of need. You cannot afford to lose focus. 100 % attention is needed, if you are to be present in the MOMENT to help in the right way.

Compassion and genuine empathy for the person's situation and their need.

Understanding that without comprehending the symptom experience and the moment by moment need, you are unlikely to be able to respond appropriately. You need to understand how you impact the person. You need to understand their symptoms and how they can be exacerbated and what that means for the person.

Flexibility so that you cannot be driven by external demands. You have to be person-centred and willing to meet each need tenderly.

Tenderness of approach makes such a difference to the person with ME, whose need is great.

This approach can be used by anyone who needs to interact with the person, visitors, friends, social workers, healthcare, professionals, family, who may need to know how to communicate, how important it is not to wear perfume, how to be flexible about visiting times, how to not feel rejected if contact is impossible, how to be willing to try again in another moment, how extra quiet and careful you need to be, given how sudden movement or actions can hurt.

What I need to know as a carer

- I need to know what to do
- I need to know when and when not to do things
- I need to know how carefully and quietly I have to perform activities and interactions
- I need to know how to communicate with the person and how they will communicate with me; it may not always be verbal
- I need to learn how to actively listen
- I need to know what affects the person negatively, what endangers health
- I need to understand the nature of the disease,

especially the dangers of pushing the person beyond their limit, however small that may seem to me
- I need to understand the risks of deterioration and how they might be triggered
- I need to understand the best way to help the person
- I need to know what is my responsibility as a carer and what is the responsibility of the person I care for
- I need to know what to say and how to say it, if I am asked to advocate for the person
- I need to know what to do in a crisis
- I need to be able to flow with the person, providing the best care in the best moment and understanding how to act at all times in the best interest of the person

(THIS CONCISE CARE GUIDE MAY BE DOWNLOADED FROM STONEBIRD : HTTPS://STONEBIRD.CO.UK/WHO.PDF)

---

1. In early studies, the discovery of elevated coxsackievirus B antibody titers in people with ME suggested enterovirus infections. Direct evidence was obtained once molecular testing methods became available. Please see this list of studies:
   https://me-pedia.org/wiki/List_of_enterovirus_infection_studies
2. The Centres for Disease Control and Prevention(CDC) state, for example that many patients with ME are sensitive to medications, especially any medication that acts on the central nervous system, such as sedating medications. They point out that therapeutic benefits can often be achieved at lower-than-standard doses. Patients with ME might tolerate or need only a fraction of the usual recommended doses for medications. After initial management with lower dosing, one or more gradual increases may be considered as necessary and as tolerated by the patient." https://www.cdc.gov/me-cfs/healthcare-providers/clinical-care-patients-mecfs/monitoring-medication.html#:~:text=Many%20patients%20with%20ME%2FCFS,lower%2Dthan%2Dstandard%20doses.

INTRODUCTION TO ESSENTIAL NOTES ON HOW TO CARE

I am very grateful to Alem Matthees and to his mother Helen Donovan, for compiling a list of care notes, based upon their own experience.

Alem requires around the clock care and hasn't left the bedroom for four and a half years.

In order to safely represent Alem and ensure his needs are met, Helen and Alem had to apply for Enduring Power of Attorney and Enduring Power of Guardianship. Without these, Helen could not fill in any forms or speak on his behalf.

It was Alem's successful legal complaint, in 2016, that resulted in the first release of anonymised data by the PACE Trial [1] researchers; a massive triumph for Alem and for the whole ME community.

I am incredibly proud to be able to include their contribution, next.

---

1. The PACE Trial:

1. Brought together (conflated) two diseases that the WHO rightly categorizes separately, neurological "ME/PVFS" (ICD-10-G93.3) and psychiatric "Fatigue Syndrome" (ICD-10-F.48.0) - and misrepresented the latter as the former.

2. Mixed at least three taxonomically different disorders in the trial cohort - those with ME/CFS (ICD-10 G93.3), even though the entry criteria exclude such patients; those with fibromyalgia (ICD- 10 M79.0) and those with a mental/behavioural disorder (ICD-10 F48.0).

3. Excluded children and those who are severely affected. The results of any trial that excluded those who are severely affected cannot be taken seriously.

4. Did not return the participants to their health or even close to it.

5. Did not study ME. For much more information on this please see my free eBook, Straightjacketed By Empty Air, page 37: https://stonebird.co.uk/emptyair/sj.pdf

ESSENTIAL NOTES ON HOW TO CARE BY ALEM MATTHEES AND HELEN DONOVAN

∾

- ME PATIENTS SHOULD HAVE the right to make choices in their life as regards to medications. Some medications can have adverse reactions and care needs to be taken when a new supplement or medication is given.
- Simple procedures to the carer, like changing sheets, clothing, should only be done when the patient is able to do this.
- Many severely ill patients are unable to tolerate noise, light and touch and it is up to the carer to be sensitive to this and at all times be respectful.
- Brushing teeth, being washed, hair combed, nails cut may not be able to be undertaken or can only be done when the patient agrees.
- Cleaning the patients room needs to be done with care and with as little disruption as possible e.g.

cleaning the carpet may need to be done with a bannister brush as a vacuum cleaner is too noisy.
- Under no circumstances should the carer insist or force the patient in any way. Stress to a severely ill ME patient is very harmful. Being stressed can cause physical reactions.
- Chemicals should be avoided as the skin is so sensitive and easily damaged.
- Healing is very slow and even rubbing can cause damage to the skin or insomnia.
- Some patients have aching muscles, joints, headaches and all over pain. The carer need to be sensitive to this.
- Many patients are unable to walk and feel hopelessly trapped and become very depressed. The carer needs to reassure the patient that they are loved and valued by the family.
- Swallowing may be an issue and the carer will need to prepare meals in a way that can be taken by the patient.
- Weight loss is a real problem and may need to be addressed by a nutritionist.
- Despite minimal activity, pain may be present in the face, on the lips (swollen lips) eye brows, jaw and all muscles.
- Deconditioning can be a serious problem.
- Cellular repair can be very difficult or non-existent.
- The carer has an enormous job in looking after a severely ill ME patient and should not feel guilty or inadequate should they seek assistance in their caring role.

51

ATTITUDES

~

Because ME is a difficult illness to understand and requires a high degree of awareness of yourself and the person's needs, there are certain attitudes that are unacceptable and need to be guarded against, when helping someone:

- Disbelief is hurtful and wrong
- Ignorance leads to misunderstanding
- Negativity makes everyone feel bad
- Unacceptance is offensive
- Impatience may exacerbate symptoms
- Judgement leads to wrong attitude
- Roughness leads to pain and distress
- Neglect means the person is not being helped
- Anger leads to disconnection and upset

- Carelessness can cause harm
- Loudness can cause pain, distress, worsening of symptoms

52

SAINT OR SINNER? CARING FULL TIME FOR SOMEONE DIAGNOSED AS HAVING VERY SEVERE ME

∼

YOUR LOVED ONE IS SUFFERING. It is coarse, raw, sweaty, smashes into shards, your fragile ego, strips naked that which you would never expose, leaves you almost unable to bear another moment of it, especially when the suffering goes on for decades without remit. Here I am learning about limits. I am learning about grief. I am learning about emotional survival. Here I cling on, feeling far out of reach, on a vicious distant edge, that few, if any, care to know about and therefore do not reach back to comfort or guide me.

[1]Suffering reeks of despair. It feels endless and hopeless. It is painful beyond description. Yet there is a pathway you must keep finding through it, in order to find meaning and restore hope. Otherwise the suffering will consume you - initially, if not long term - unless you can find a way to see all, including loss and grief, as a path and somehow find crucial self-support and milestones to help you measure along the way.

Then you can find that it is possible to face your situation with dignity, you can find meaning and purpose, even in the most awful, indescribable circumstances and desolation even.

I am particularly inspired by Viktor Frankl, a survivor from Auschwitz. He confirms for me that you can attain spiritual comfort, meaning and insight from the most desperate of moments: that is his burning message and challenge, that helps me whilst living through seemingly endless, continual losses that never completely resolve, as I live and care full time for my wife, who is profoundly ill and disabled and has borne indescribable suffering for decades. Who has any idea, who could possibly comprehend the innumerable losses we have both suffered?

Freedom of movement is a significant loss. You can go out, but you have to go without the person you might want to be with. This is an adjustment. Not as wanted, expected, needed, hoped for. People do not see you the same way. You might be a couple, but you are a couple without the presence of your partner, if they are homebound.

You, the care-giver, you have a choice every day to make. The option to go out, to be involved externally in other things, do the ordinary things in the community that others are engaged with, is a constant possibility, even if you do not feel inclined to follow it. Your own confinement to the house is a choice, made purely by your decision to provide care for the one you love, though it may not always feel like a choice for some, but might feel at times more of an obligation, an expectation, a necessary need to be met.

There is a loss of sharing in the moment, even if you can include the person by videoing events or describing the experience in conversation afterwards, it is nowhere the same as being together, sharing a moment, being seen publicly as a couple or a family. Often people, you find, are ignorant in how they just shut out the other missing person from the event or the conversation. That is unbearably painful initially, then it becomes an emotional pain, a loss, a gnawing grief that resides deep inside, not necessarily recognised or obvious.

> The person not talked about or acknowledged, can become the 'elephant in the room' or even no 'elephant' at all, simply extinct to all intent.

Visitors may seem not to realise your own stress level. The ongoing distress of providing a high burden of physical or emotional care seems completely invisible to them. You appear to be some kind of saintly, giving person, expected to give to them and entertain them too, without recognition of your own need to be looked after. Others, in our experience, either look down upon you, insult, negate, offend you, criticise you or patronise you. We have literally had garbage dumped on us, cleared out rubbish from a garage that someone did not want the inconvenience of taking to the dump, thinking it was some sort of charity.

You are not seen for who you are often; there is a distorted view of you, either as saint or sinner. Neither is accurate, balanced, whole. There is a loss of perspective and perception of you.

You are especially a saint to those who could not imagine doing what you do, who perhaps cannot deal with others vulnerability, frailty or need, perhaps, particularly for these many decades, maybe through feelings of inadequacy, disinterest even or just having different values.

> You are most certainly a sinner, when you start to fail to comply with other people's demands and expectations of you, especially when you begin to miss family and social engagements repeatedly and when you put the care need of your loved one, necessarily, before them.

You are also treated like a sinner by others who make false judgments about your role and see you as someone who is somehow inferior, scrounging, not deserving of respect or equal value, not actually 'working'. They have no idea about what you do, how stressed or stretched you are, how skilled care-giving is, how essential your role.

I am seen as both.

And so you lead a double life, one also invisible to a large degree from normal life and normal lives. You too disappear, to a degree, change the way you live, adjust to a new way of being housebound often yourself. The losses you accept are different to the person who is ill, but there are still many losses that you share together as well as ones unique to you, that you need to deal with repeatedly, in order to survive and more than that, find that your life, as Viktor Frankl says, has the most profound meaning and value.

---

1. Who can possibly imagine living in such an assaulting and broken world for decades, without adequate investigation, care or support?
    - We receive no support from the Church or local community
    - We have had been forced to live below the poverty line
    - Society has lost out on our professional skills (I am an award-winning Nurse, my wife is a qualified Social Worker, Counsellor and Teacher)
    - We live in almost complete isolation, as my wife's agony and hypersensitivities are so intense, that she cannot bear contact or interaction
    - We have not been able to have children of our own

- I was in my 30's when my wife became ill, shortly after we got married, I am now in my 60's
- We were both highly respected professionals, but I have openly been called a "waste of space" as a carer
- My wife's profound suffering goes unrecognised and ignored as if she does not exist
- Nieces and nephews have grown into adulthood, married, had children who we do not know and who do not know us
- Parents have got old and people have gotten sick without being able to visit them even when dying or to attend their funerals

We live in a hamlet, four miles from what is regularly voted the best beach in England. My wife has never even seen it, let alone put her feet in the endless sand, felt the sea splash over her toes, heard the pines whisper above the dunes.

https://meassociation.org.uk/2019/08/very-severe-me-its-time-for-something-new-by-greg-crowhurst-16-august-2019/

53

PARTNERSHIP

Partnership is not just about care, but about a way of being with the person to enhance their life and minimise the sense of isolation and separation they may feel due to the severity of illness.

Its aim is to find peaceful flowing moments that reach beyond or through the illness, to connect with the person and touch their lives with goodness so that your life may also be touched with goodness in return.

You appreciate who the person is. Partnership is not just one sided, but a mutually rewarding experience based on respect and relationship, where both lives are enhanced by the connection.

A 'partnership model[1]' stands in contrast to a so-called 'dominator model' of social organisation: one which is based upon social ranking: typically authoritarian and top-down. (Eisler 1995).

A posture of partnership represents a 'paradigm shift' (Kuhn 1970[2]), a change in our fundamental assumptions about reality.

Rather than 'power over', a partnership perspective is concerned with 'power from within, power to enable ourselves and others to achieve the ends we desire.' (Montouri & Conti p.20[3])

Partnership requires two way connectedness, an acceptance of equality of personhood both of the carer and the person needing care. In Severe and Very Severe ME the illness can so easily get in the way of seeing this, from both sides; a determination to grow in positive regard and respect is needed, although that can be difficult given the intensity of physical suffering and the stress of the moment.

Co-operation is key to good caring. That must be mutual to avoid harm, disconnection, mistrust and misinterpretation of events.

A partnership approach requires a commitment to grow together and work out how to help, when to help and when to wait. What to do and what not to do. When to try now and when to try later, but never to walk away and neglect or give up.

It needs input from both sides, no matter how long that takes to gain and how complicated the communication is.

How to help someone with Severe ME is not necessarily obvious or apparent, it is complex, particularly because of the high risk of deterioration from seemingly small interventions. The specific experience of each person needs to be learned and understood as much as possible, because each person will be different in what they can tolerate and when and how they can be helped. You need to be able to read the signs very carefully.

Knowing how and when to engage is often unpredictable because of the illness and its impact and the post-exertional experience. In the absence of clear signs, you have to be intuitive and empathic and always learn from every mistake you make.

It is almost impossible to comprehend the chaos the person's body is experiencing from different factors; noise, light, touch, colours, chemicals, movement, perfume as well as the illness itself, your very presence in their environment, the effort required to engage with you, all can be too much for the person to deal with, in any one moment.

The person might appear to be coping, until you try to help; just you entering into their space can tip the balance for the worse, unexpectedly and unintentionally.

Nothing is simple and straight forward in Severe ME; always remember that you are entering into a world of chaos, where everything is turned upside down and not as expected, where everything in the environment, including yourself, is potentially hostile and harmful without meaning to be.

It requires infinite flexibility on your part to be open to stopping everything and what you might judge as doing nothing apparently useful or worthwhile other than just being with the person; focused on how you can make a difference:

With an open heart: you bring compassion, sensitivity, valuing and respect.

With an open posture: you bring acceptance, warmth, focus and attention.

With an open mind:

- You are not closed in your thinking about Severe and Very Severe ME.
- You are open to partnership, to working it out together.
- You are open to growing in awareness.
- You are open to understanding the reality of the person.

- You are open to learning how to do things differently.
- You are open to changing the things that you get wrong and you are able to admit you might not always get it right, as it is complex.
- You are open to entering into the other person's experience.

---

1. For much more background on Partnership theory and practice please see: https://stonebird.co.uk/dissertation.html
2. Kuhn T (1970) 'The Structure of Scientific Revolutions' University of Chicago Press in Montuori & Conti 1993 p. 7
3. Montuori A & Conti I (1993) 'From Power to Partnership, Creating the Future of Love, Work and Community.' (San Francisco, Haper)

54

WHAT WRONG ASSUMPTIONS CAN YOU EASILY MAKE

∼

It is very easy to make the following wrong assumptions if you do not recognise how physically fragile, vulnerable or weak the person diagnosed with Severe or Very Severe ME is.

Wrong assumptions:

1. "The person is just asleep", when either they are too weak to communicate or are physically paralysed, yet internally conscious.

This is a basic error of judgement. It is not easy to tell the difference, but to the person paralysed yet needing support, to be left alone under the assumption that they are resting or asleep can be very frustrating or upsetting.

Action required: It takes time and attention to know how to approach this situation, so a plan of how to manage this situation can be individually worked out.

2. "I have to do this by myself."

No, you are always in a two-way interaction, even when the other person is unable to communicate with you. What you say and what you do and how you respond make all the difference in the world.

Action required: Taking time to learn about individual symptoms and your own impact upon them is essential. Developing an understanding that you are in partnership with the other person, helps tremendously.

3. "I can do what I want, when I want, how I want, if the person cannot see me."

No, if a person is particularly hypersensitive, then your actions anywhere in the home can or may impact the person negatively.

Action required: Be aware that any noise anywhere in the home may still be heard by the person who has acute noise sensitivity, even if you do not think that you are being overly noisy. Footsteps on stairs make a thud, shutting doors or cupboards can bang very loudly, switching on a kettle, running a tap in the bathroom or kitchen can be a torment. Make sure you shut all doors carefully, pull all curtains across the doors if they are needed. It might help to agree in principle what can be tolerated and when and where it might be best to do things that require some noise. Remember that however quiet you think you are, silence means no noise.

4. "If I put my head phones on, while I do the washing up or other tasks, then I won't be noisy."

Wrong, if you put headphones on you may be able to enjoy listening to music etc while you do a task, but there is still likely to be some sound coming out of the headphones, leaking into the environment which may still cause irritation. If you have head phones on, then you cannot judge how quiet or noisy you are being whilst doing the task itself. If you wear headphones, you will not be able to hear the other person trying to communicate with you that you are making too much noise.

Action required: Only wear headphones if you have agreed it with the person and it will not cause problems for them or risk deteriorating their health.

People can easily go without things because you missed the moment to notice their need or they were unable to try and communicate more than once.

Do try not to squander the persons very limited energy and ability.

5. "I just want to finish what I am doing before I go and help the person."

No, timing is everything in supporting people severely disabled with ME. If you get the wrong moment, the energy or ability to tolerate the action needed, may be lost.

Action required: *If* you are asked to do something, then make sure your response is quick and careful. Do not leave a person unnecessarily long, needing a drink or wanting help to go to the toilet, for example. If they then cannot manage the thing that they needed and asked for help with, because you were preoccupied with something that you could have easily left, then the person may suffer as a consequence.

Care must be a priority. Understanding how small the window of opportunity may be for the person to engage with you is important, in order to try and get care right. Respond efficiently and respectfully.

6. "Because I can't hear it, it isn't there."

No, if a person says that they can hear a noise, believe them. It may be tormenting them, due to increased hypersensitivities and acute hearing.

You may be able to block out external sounds that the person cannot.

A sound may seem much louder to the other person than to how you are experiencing it. Sound can be extremely irritating, painful to excruciating and exposure, even to what seems like tiny noise, unexpected or repeated noises or very loud noise can be devastating and deteriorative.

Action required: If the person experiences Hyperacusis take time to learn what that means specifically for them. Severity can vary from time to time or person to person. Become as aware as possible of new external noises that might be a threat to the person's health and well being. Always accept that a sound is an issue for the person if they say it is. Do not consider yourself the best judge.

7. "Because I can't smell it, it isn't there."

People may have increased sensitivity to perfume and chemicals. You may not notice this yourself. You may be accustomed to certain smells or even like them or find them pleasant or neutral.

To the person whose health deteriorates from such exposure, it is devastating if they are not believed or their reality downplayed or minimised. It can be a major issue if you come into the home having absorbed perfume from the outside environment or put perfume on or used perfumed products inadvertently. Symptoms of allergy can be very scary or unpleasant.

Action required: Never argue that you don't smell of perfume because you are not aware of it. Follow any procedures such as showering, changing clothes etc., use non-perfumed products yourself, that you have agreed with the person. This may feel like an unnecessary over reaction or a hassle in your busy day, but it is so important in order to keep the person safe. Always believe them, don't debate. This can be very damaging to relationship and trust.

8. "I will just do this tiny thing that I want to do, because I will be so quick that the person will not notice, so it can't really hurt."

For the person who is very severely ill and hypersensitive, every thing you say or do in their vicinity or in their home impacts them in ways that you will never be able to truly comprehend. Any unexpected exposure to noise, light, movement in their space, that has not been agreed, can be catastrophic.

Action required: Be aware that that little thing, that barely makes a sound to you, can still risk triggering deterioration and unnecessary extra suffering. You can literally ruin someone's day because you wanted to pick up something you felt that you needed in that wrong moment, thinking you could get away with the seemingly slight noise or movement it would take to get it, disregarding the other's reality, just for a moment.

> Learn patience and tolerance. Be person-centred not self-centred. Be as aware as possible of the other person and how everything you do impacts them.

CARER SKILLS

If you get the approach wrong, be aware that you can literally ruin hours, days, weeks, months, years of a person's life, by unintentionally causing massive deterioration.

Some useful/important skills to develop

Communication skills:

- Being able to listen when the person cannot enunciate clearly. The person may not be able to speak clearly due to weakness, partial paralysis, lack of energy.
- Being able to understand limited language. As energy runs out words may disappear from the person's mental access.
- Being able to understand the meaning of words

used. Sometimes the wrong word may be used or words may be switched around unintentionally.
- Being able to learn a particular sign language or way of communicating. Some people may lose their voice temporarily or longer term.
- Being able to use alternative methods of communication. This may be the only way a person can convey their needs.
- Being able to recognise when a person is running out of energy by their deteriorating language skills. Mental effort uses as much energy as physical effort.
- Being able to communicate safely with the person so that they are not overloaded by too many words. Too many words together can overload the mind and be difficult or painful to process.
- Being able to not speak too fast. If sentences are spoken too quickly, they may be impossible to comprehend and lead to deterioration.
- Being able to tailor information. Mental overload can lead to shut down and an inability to tolerate more information or communicate at all.
- Being able to speak not too loudly. The loudness of voice is magnified unimaginably and painfully if the person has hyperacusis (noise sensitivity) and may trigger symptom deterioration which then stops all possibility of communication.
- Being able to find out information without asking direct questions, for example, by making an observation as opposed to a direct question. Questions may be too difficult for the person to tolerate or literally too painful to retrieve the answers to.

- Being able to judge appropriate distance, not too close to the person or too far away. Distance can affect communication negatively or positively, depending on how well the person can tolerate you near them, how loudly they may be able to speak, if at all, how much effort is then required to be heard or how tolerable the level of your voice is depending on distance.
- Being able to not gesticulate wildly when speaking. Movement may trigger massive symptom deterioration, confusion, disorientation, irritability.
- Being able to recognise when to speak and when to be silent and wait. Timing and awareness are everything.
- Being able to know how to speak appropriately, if asked, on behalf of the person. You need to represent accurately their message, not your interpretation of it, which may not be quite the same.
- Being able to read subtle changes in facial expression and body language. There is a pressing need to avoid overstimulation and deterioration.
- Being able to be to be supportive and affirming. Your energy can have a dramatic effect if you are irritated, tired, over exuberant or dismissive or even be negating, though unintentionally.
- Knowing how to enable someone else to safely be with the person. The person needs to be safely communicated with in the correct way by everyone they have to engage with.
- Being able to advocate. The person might be relying on you to speak on their behalf to keep them safe.

- Being able to cope with changing emotions. Emotional lability is a recognised aspect of ME.

Practical Skills

- Knowing not to do the wrong thing at the wrong moment. You need to know where the person is, how they are, what they can tolerate in any moment to avoid deterioration.
- Being able to learn the specific way each task needs to be done for a specific person's needs and symptom experience. Each person is individual and has specific symptoms and needs in relation to them.
- Being able to do things extremely quietly or to plan to do things that are difficult to tolerate, away from the person at the right time. To ignore sound or light or movement sensitivity or other symptoms is to risk serious deterioration and the relationship breaking down.
- Being able to perform tasks efficiently. The need is immediate and great, often.
- Being able to be flexible. Things are not always tolerable or achievable, the right moment must be found.
- Being gentle in your actions. It is important to be aware how sensitive and frail the person might be.
- Being aware of the person at all times that you are in their presence. To not notice how you are impacting the person can be catastrophic.
- Being able to learn how to do things together at the pace of the other person. The person needs you to

slow your energy and pace, to flow with them to get the need met.
- Being able to follow instructions absolutely, to do what you are asked. To not do so is to negate the person, who knows what they need, when and how they need it and cannot do it without you, but needs it done in a specific and tolerable way.
- Being able to help with memory. Cognitive dysfunction can impact remembering important information and needs.
- Aware cooking skills. You may need to make specific food in specific ways for dietary needs.
- Aware cleaning skills. Cleaning is a major challenge around someone with multiple environmental hypersensitivities, in pain or with limited energy and needs to be done carefully, quietly, attentively when tolerable.
- Aware unpacking skills. Unpacking things is noisy and access to things needs considering when putting things away to ensure accessibility if possible or required.
- Aware food preparation skills. Food and drinks may need to be prepared with only specific ingredients due to hypersensitivities and multiple chemical sensitivity may need to be considered in the way things are prepared.

Personal Care Skills

- Being able to learn how to lift and help transfer safely if required, this needs great awareness and training to avoid hurting yourself or the person.

- Being able to learn how to work safely in low light if required, this needs careful consideration for both of you.
- Being able to act carefully and quietly with no sudden, unexpected movements, this is particularly so for someone with movement and/or noise sensitivity to reduce risk of deterioration.
- Being able to follow any necessary routine and provide familiarity, security and safety in the way care and interaction is provided.
- Being very good at time keeping. If things need doing at specific times, waiting is very difficult trying to hold on to a moment of possibility and limited energy, that may be dissipating, the longer the wait required.
- Being able to learn to help a person eat and drink in the right way for them. It requires skilled input and a high level of awareness, to safely help someone eat or drink and avoid choking.
- Being available and ready to help when needed, this is absolutely essential because nothing is predictable or necessarily repeatable or tolerable.
- Knowing the best way to approach a person. This requires concern, interest, intention, determination, sensitivity and a willingness to learn.
- Knowing the best way to convey your presence without causing shock or confusion. How you approach, when you approach and how you announce your presence to the person are extremely important, because the wrong way can be traumatic, shocking, deteriorative, painful.
- Being able to learn spacial awareness around the

person, being aware where they are, in relation to any activity you might be undertaking. It is so important that you understand and know how you impact the person, even if you are not in the same room.
- Knowing how to help the person wash and care for other personal needs with dignity and safety. It is a vulnerable experience for the person and requires great sensitivity and careful action, to help them not feel demeaned, embarrassed or disrespected.

Personal Awareness Skills

- Being able to walk carefully, quietly, consciously.
- Being able to learn what might be a specific hazard for the person: things that are noisy ie clocks, alarms, phone ring/vibrating. Activities that are noisy ie cooking, cutting up food, putting shopping away. Things that might unduly expose the person to light ie computer/ phone screens. Things that might cause too much pressure or pain ie clothes, bedding. Things that might involve sudden movement, like a video, a dog wagging its tail, the hands of a clock, moving too close by the person. Things that might create a chemical hazard or perfume hazards, pertinent to the persons hypersensitivity.
- Learning to be aware of possible pressure points on the body, skin, nose with glasses, shoes too tight etc, because pressure sensitivity may be severe and the slightest unexpected thing can cause harm without realising the risk.

- Being aware of immediate and wider environmental hazards, such as building work, lawnmowers, alarm bells etc. The wider environment needs protection against as much as possible and you need to take avoiding action if possible.
- Knowing how to dress so that the person is not impacted by sound of material or colour, pattern, brightness. You may not naturally be aware how noisy your clothes are when you walk or put an item of clothing on or how irritating, painful or confusing a pattern or bright colour might be to the person, but you need to learn how this impacts, to ensure that you do not not unnecessarily trigger worsening of symptoms or cause extra difficulty tolerating you in the room.
- Being able to maintain focus on a task, to avoid doing something wrong. If you do not notice what you are doing or if you do not notice something important, the need will not necessarily be met safely or properly and trust can be broken.
- Being willing to reflect and grow in your learning: how to help or be with the person in the best way. The more natural things become, the better you can flow with the person and the better the persons experience overall will be and the safer they will feel with you providing their care, hopefully.

Qualities That Help:

- Patience
- Kindness
- Warmth

- Willingness to understand
- Openness to learn
- Openness to listen
- Openness to work with the person
- Sensitivity
- Flexibility
- Acceptance
- Enough Energy
- Ability to reach out
- Empathy
- Respect
- Honesty
- Integrity
- Dexterity
- Willingness to wait
- Comfortable in silence
- Comfortable with stillness
- Non-judgmental approach
- Confidence
- Genuineness
- Sense of equality of personhood
- Creativity
- Valuing
- Validating
- Enabling
- Empowering

56

A MIND/BODY/EMOTION/SPIRIT APPROACH

When approaching a care issue, it can help to take a Mind, Body, Spirit, Emotion approach. Below are a few questions that might aid you in your reflection.

MIND:

- What am I thinking about when I approach the person with Severe or Very Severe ME?
- Can I focus solely about what I am doing?
- Have I thought ahead about what potential issues might come up to deal with?
- Do I understand that ME is an organic, physical disease, with multi-system dysfunction?
- Do I have the knowledge or experience that I need to perform the tasks that I need to do?

BODY:

- Am I able to be gentle enough, when I help the person?
- Am I too tired to help sensitively and carefully?
- Am I in pain anywhere myself or feeling unwell?
- Am I strong enough to perform all the tasks required?

SPIRIT:

- How do I feel about being with the person?
- Can I connect with the person and their need?
- Am I flowing with the right energy to have contact with the person?
- Do I understand, as best as possible, how the symptoms affect the person in getting their need met and what care I need to take in order to flow with the person?
- Am I aware and alert?

EMOTION:

- What is my emotional state?
- How are my emotions going to impact upon my interaction?

- Am I distracted about other issues?
- Am I emotionally available?

57

DO NO HARM

IT IS TOO EASY to trigger deterioration in someone with Very Severe ME, by the simplest action, wrongly timed or inappropriately carried out. Because of the complex multi-system dysfunction and extreme hypersensitivity that they experience, people with Severe and Very Severe ME do not respond in the same way as in other illnesses.

> You can help or harm. There is no room for carelessness, clumsiness, impatience, inattention; the harm you can inadvertently do to a person with Very Severe ME is not just in the immediate moment; the impact may go on for days, weeks, months and can be catastrophic.

You need to make sure that you are fully aware, that you know that ME is a serious and severe neurological disease. The person you are about to interact with needs specific, sensitive physical support and assistance. Your main aim should be to make sure that they get the physical help they require, on their terms.

You need to make sure that the thoughts you have are the right thoughts to have in order to engage with someone with ME. If you believe that the person just needs encouragement or can do more, if pushed, you could do great harm.

> You have to do more than your best to limit any harm to the person with Severe or Very Severe ME. You must care about how you are caring.

Care, of itself, will not be enough, unless it is grounded in a true appreciation of the nightmare reality you can create by getting it wrong. You have to take care of the fine details of caring as well as the basic care needs. It is not just what you do; it is how you do it and in which moment you do it. In Severe and Very Severe ME, it is the acute nature of the harm that can be done by the smallest thing, that you need to understand and really care about.

Caring does not take place in a vacuum. If you get it wrong it is disastrous, but if you repeatedly get it wrong you damage the relationship and trust that you have with the person. There is a power issue, where you hold a lot of power as a carer. You must not take advantage of that power or misinterpret the person, because of your inadequacy at comprehending their need and how to safely meet it.

There is no place for complacency, mediocrity or carelessness in the life of someone with Very Severe ME. Whatever you do, right or wrong, make sure you learn what helps and what hurts.

Make a commitment to always do better and always intend to get it right! Know exactly what you are doing and be prepared, even so you may not always be able to predict a bad reaction. Stop what you are doing immediately and wait till re-engagement is possible. Follow any agreed protocols.

If the indications are that the person is suffering, distressed and not flowing with you, never keep on doing something because you think you are right.

The person who is severely ill will always know better than you what impact you are having upon them and what they can tolerate. Always wait and listen.

Learn how to interpret their reaction and communication. Never leave the person feeling bad about themselves because you got it wrong.

HOW TO APPROACH SOMEONE WITH SEVERE OR VERY SEVERE ME: A QUICK CHECK LIST

- With caution
- With knowledge
- With gentle attention
- With no wrong assumption
- With an open heart
- With an open mind
- With due care
- With the best understanding possible
- With sensitivity
- With patience
- With a willingness to listen
- With recognition of the need to be attentive
- With the intention to be responsive
- With an attitude of equality of personhood
- With awareness
- With a person-centred focus
- With no judgement
- Without demand or undue expectation

59

HOW TO HELP THE PERSON WITH SEVERE OR VERY SEVERE ME

∼

- Listen to them.
- Believe them.
- Ask them how they are, if possible.
- Talk with them about their lives, if able.
- Validate them.
- Learn about the illness so that you understand how seriously ill a person with Severe ME actually is.
- Show concern for them.
- Acknowledge that you see how truly physically ill they are.
- Take account of their hypersensitivities.
- Be aware of what makes them more ill.
- Be aware of how loud you talk or how much you talk or how much movement you make and do not wear perfumed products. All these things can have a positive or negative impact.

- Speak up for people with ME.
- Challenge wrong thinking in others.
- Challenge wrong beliefs and attitudes.
- Lobby the government for better health equality for people with ME.
- Demand a proper definition be used to identify neurological ME and separate it from fatigue illnesses.
- Understand the politics of ME and the vested interests underlying the neglect.
- Keep in touch with the person in what ever way you know they can tolerate.
- Understand how difficult communication is and accommodate their needs.
- Offer to help in ways that really will help them, not make them more ill.
- Show them that you understand how sad it is for them and you, that they cannot engage in normal life.
- Invite them to social gatherings even if they cannot go, include them by remembering them at family events but do not make them feel obliged to attend or guilty of refusal.
- Take photos for them, remember they still belong, even if the illness keeps them separate.
- Make them still feel part of the family even though they are forced to be absent because of illness.
- Do not assume that they are not interested or do not care because they are not with you enjoying things together anymore or cannot write or ring or answer the phone.

- See how isolated they are and keep connected when possible in a way that works for them.
- Offer genuinely helpful practical support.
- Buy presents that are suitable for the person taking into account their hypersensitivity particularly to materials, food, and chemicals and anything else you know about.
- Be aware that the media can sometimes misrepresent people with ME. Write complaints about it if possible and challenge misrepresentation. Don't believe it.
- Help people to have their illness treated fairly and equally as a physical disease, with adequate testing and properly funded and identified research for ME rather than CFS.
- Understand the difference and make a difference in people's lives.

WHAT DOES BEING PRESENT ACTUALLY MEAN, FOR PEOPLE WITH COMPLEX SYMPTOM EXPERIENCE AND HYPERSENSITIVITY?

∽

IT IS NOT SIMPLE, nor does it even, necessarily, feel reasonable or possible sometimes, yet the ability to be fully present lies at the heart of effective care.

> Being present is so much more than just being in the room with the person. To be in the room without awareness of what it means to be truly present, can be catastrophic and deteriorative - the very opposite of your intention.

In order to be truly present you need to focus on the person:

- Understand the symptoms that they are experiencing and how they affect the person directly - what level of suffering they might be experiencing

which may get in the way of connecting and two way interaction.
- Recognise the signs of deterioration, increased agony and any likely triggers for worsening their experience.
- Be aware of your own inner energy and external non-verbal communication and body language.
- If you are irritated, disinterested, distracted, unmotivated, feeling critical, worried, sad, preoccupied or negative yourself, for whatever reason, unfortunately the person is likely to sense this and feel exhausted, irritated, disturbed, negated, tormented and may be deteriorated by it.
- Be patient and still in yourself, especially if the person has severe movement or noise sensitivity. Even the slightest, most seemingly insignificant noise or sudden even subtle movement, can do unimaginable harm, depending on the severity of symptoms.
- Be quiet, but make sure that quiet is peaceful, not agitated by your own energy.
- Wait for the right moment.
- If you remain in the room it will mean standing or sitting in silence, noticing how the person is, being ready to help at the right moment.
- It does not mean read a book or play a video game or twiddle your fingers, tap your foot impatiently or unawarely or write emails, look at interesting websites, use an app; unless the person has said they can specifically tolerate such things and it is ok to do so.
- Know how and when to respond without being told.

Know how important it is to be ready to help, to be able to do things in the right way.
- Look for the right moment to communicate or move.

All this is just the minimum required for anyone wanting to provide sensitive aware care.

> You see, if you can achieve or convey a sense of harmony, peace and being together, even in the most desperate moments, the outcome can be one of flow and togetherness through the tremendous suffering caused by the illness.

The sense of utter total isolation can be broken and the relationship can only be strengthened by such congruence and compassion.

Being truly present then, is an affirming experience that conveys a message to the person that you know how to be with them, that you are aware of how difficult it is for them to tolerate your presence.

Without it, disconnection can occur and the whole experience of meeting need and the flow that comes from being together in aware partnership, becomes harder to achieve or sustain.

PRESENCE EXPERIENCED AS PHYSICAL TOUCH, BY CHRISTINE FENTON

WE NEED TO FIND a way for people to 'get' that physical presence is experienced as physical touch:

- the closer the presence the harder the touch
- the faster the presence the faster the touch
- the louder the presence the sharper the touch

Close, fast, loud presence translates to a body needing to withdraw from pain, intense pressured pain with intermittent shards of glass internally through the veins, muscles, brain, all going on at the same time, but the body can't withdraw, it can only endure until the presence leaves.

62

CARING FOR SOMEONE DIAGNOSED WITH SEVERE OR VERY SEVERE ME, THE NEED TO BE STRONG

> *It's her worse nightmare and it's your worse nightmare too."* Greg Crowhurst, **"Seventh Circle of Hell"** https://www.youtube.com/watch?v=y6TkTHLQjIk

You need to be strong because not enough people are speaking out about the truth of this serious neurological disease. It is very, very hard when you are isolated or hidden and not seen or you have no energy or limited physical ability to speak up for yourself.

You have to be strong because the anger and despair, at the neglect and isolation, are hard to bear.

Almost every path is blocked to the person with ME. There are very few consultants who can really help. You have to find a safe doctor, one who knows that ME is a neurological disease, with multi-system dysfunction; it sounds simple, but in practice many people with Severe and Very Severe ME do not even have this.

You have to try and find a way to deal with all the complex

emotions, caring for someone with Severe or Very Severe ME brings up in you; it can be a lonely path.

Family and friends fall by the wayside, not understanding your reality or the extraordinary pressures on you as a carer. Often you have to choose between living in the world, engaged in normal social roles and interactions or being with the person with Severe or Very Severe ME, who can no longer be a part of all that.

It is a painful choice.

There are very few who see how stressed and distressed the carer is. Those that do might even get into being divisive or blaming the person with Severe/Very Severe ME for taking you away from them. You get tired. It is hard work and still people do not understand; which is demoralising.

> Very few stand by you. The ones who know, because they are going through it themselves are often too exhausted and necessarily focused on the one they are caring for, dealing with their own hurts and exhaustion, to support or encourage you; though they do when they can.

Broad shoulders are required to bear the other's never ending suffering, the incapacitating weight of inertia, the need to keep pushing for change.

To be strong is to be in touch with your own centre, your feelings, your values. To be strong is to be your own person.

To be strong is to know what you stand for and to come from that position.

To be strong is to be able to see and name the truth for what it is, that matters so much in Severe and Very Severe ME.

To be strong is to be able to stand back from the situation

you are in and recognise the awful, raging, devastating symptoms that are causing the person you care for such distress or inability to even tolerate your presence.

Strength in this situation is the courage to try and see the world from the perspective of someone with Severe/Very Severe ME; not that you can even get close to it.

What can make all the difference between the person having their needs met and nothing being done, is your ability to recognise the need and take the initiative to do something about it.

To be strong is to take responsibility, to act, without needing always to be told what to do, yet to act always with integrity, always with the greatest care and respect.

Perhaps the greatest strength of all lies in being able to pick yourself up. Even if it is only the hope that is left in your heart, to still find great meaning and infinite purpose in your day.

A QUICK ALPHABET OF POINTS FOR CARERS

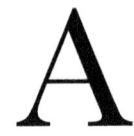

A

- ADVOCACY: if you are asked to advocate for the person, make sure you accurately and adequately represent them.
- ASK: if you do not know what to do, ask the person at an appropriate time or whoever the person agrees you can ask. Avoid panic and ignorance.
- ATTENTION: pay attention to the smallest details. Pay attention to any signals the person may be giving out non- verbally as well as verbally.
- AWARENESS: develop a conscious awareness of the person and their needs. Be aware of how every

sound, movement, action you make, impacts the person.

B

- BE CAREFUL: it is easy to make a mistake. Every action can lead to catastrophe potentially, if done wrongly.
- BELIEVE: believe in the person and accept their illness, even if you do not fully understand it.
- Bold: be bold in your actions and believe in yourself as a carer. Get it right.

C

- CALM: remain calm, even if a problem or crisis arises. Calmness aids right action.
- CARE: care enough to really learn all you can about the person's needs and issues, so that you can care safely for the person, even when communication is difficult or impossible.
- CAUTIOUS: be cautious in your actions around the person, especially when you are getting to know them. Only do what you are asked.
- CONCERN: concern yourself with the health and wellbeing of the person so that you can notice tiny changes in energy and ability to tolerate your presence and the help needed.
- CONFIDENCE: perform tasks confidently, as fear or anxiety can lead to mistakes and uncertainty.
- CONSCIOUS: consciously carry out your actions and care tasks so that accidents and mistakes do not

occur and so that you are aware of how the person is, in any moment.
- CREATIVE: creative solutions are often needed, as needs are complex and answers not always obvious or easy to find.

D

- DELIBERATE: any task you are given will have a deliberate need, even if it is not clear to you why things need doing in a particular way. It is best to follow any deliberate instructions, not think you can do things easier or better, without checking.
- DELICATELY: when people are extremely sensitive, they need a delicate approach, to ensure that they do not come to harm or deteriorate unintentionally.
- DILIGENCE: diligence is required at all times as mistakes can have long term affect and also result in a lack of confidence.

E

- EASE: in time you will hopefully learn to flow with ease, if you persevere in getting things right with the person.
- EFFECTIVE: it is important to be effective in all you do. No half hearted approaches will suffice.
- EFFICIENT: the person may not be able to tolerate much contact, so the most efficient way of helping is most important.
- EFFORT: make the effort to learn about Severe and Very Severe ME, to understand the person's needs

and reactions, to really comprehend how the person communicates and feels.
- EMOTION: be aware of how your emotional state can affect the person because they are extra sensitive.
- EXPERIENCE: experience, with time, brings knowledge.

F

- FLEXIBLE: you need to be willing to help in a flexible fashion at the moment that the person can tolerate or engage with you, you need to be willing to stop or go away if asked or return later if necessary or wait patiently till the right moment presents itself.
- FLOW: it is important to flow with the person rather than block or drain their extremely limited energy. More will be achieved if you can flow with the person, not against them or pressured by external demands.
- FOCUSED: when helping it is important to focus on what you are doing and be aware of how this affects the person. You may have to focus on specific needs for safety. Develop a habit of focussing on what is required.
- FRIENDLY: having a friendly manner eases tension and hopefully does not use up extra energy relating to you and dealing with your presence.

G

- GENTLE: aim to be gentle in your contact with the

person. Gentle energy is more likely to be tolerated generally.
- GENUINE: a genuine relationship between you, built on trust and working in partnership, is most likely to bring the greatest rewards for you both.

H

- HARM: harm can easily result from wrong thought or action or even from just doing the right thing in the wrong moment. Be careful to avoid accidental or unintentional harm.
- HARSH: a harsh voice or reaction can affect the symptoms of the person negatively. Be careful how you speak and when you speak and notice how you feel.
- HELPFUL: it helps if you genuinely feel helpful in what you are doing, if you want to be there for the person.
- HONOURABLE: approaching caring with honour inspires the highest values and trust.
- HOPEFUL: approach the person hopefully. Negative energy or upset can be catastrophic, as any emotion that you experience can have an affect.

I

- IGNORANCE: is unacceptable when caring for a person with Severe/Very severe ME, because so much harm can inadvertently be done, just doing ordinary things wrongly timed, too loudly or carelessly with ignorance. Make sure you know what you need to know to keep caring safe. Deliberate ignorance is when you have been told, but chose to ignore the information you have been given about the person. That is completely unacceptable.

J

- JOYFUL: it can be a joyful experience when everything flows in harmony.

K

- KINDNESS: kindness is key to success if it is rooted in genuine values and principles of care. Kindness must be about meeting the needs of the person, not just feeling good about yourself, thinking you are a kind person, but still getting things wrong. Kindness is not enough without sound knowledge and good practice.

L

- LEARNING: is essential. It is important to keep learning and growing and constantly aiming to get it right and make the persons life work better for your involvement with them.
- LISTEN: listen for clues and be aware of changes and issues that might arise. Listen to the persons communication on every level, verbal and non-
- verbal and learn to respond appropriately.

M

- MINDFULNESS: a mindful approach, calm and open, not fearful or anxious, is required to flow as well as possible with the person and their needs.
- MOMENT: a moment approach, flowing with awareness of when and how to perform a task or interact is often the most helpful way of attending to a person diagnosed with Severe or Very Severe ME. It is not possible to predict how a person will be, moment to moment, therefore you may have to wait often for the right moment.

N

- NEGATIVITY: is unhelpful and makes it harder to help the person. It will most likely increase stress in yourself and block energy, can even impact health negatively.

O

- OPEN: be open to grow and learn new ways of being and doing things.

P

- PARTNERSHIP: means working out how to help and when and what to do, in partnership with the person. It is based on equality of personhood.
- PATIENCE: patience is required every day, as helping

a person with complex health and care issues and hypersensitivities, who will experience a post-exertional reaction, makes life and caring somewhat unpredictable and this can be frustrating. Patience then is essential in approaching the person and every task, whether day or night.
- PREPARED: be prepared in advance for as many potential difficult circumstances and problems in advance as possible, so that you know what to do even if the person is unable to speak and tell you.

Q

- QUIETLY: it is most likely that the person you help will have some degree of noise sensitivity, some more, some less, some profound. Some may be able to use ear protection to help reduce the harm from noise but others may not. It is important to approach all tasks and movements, then, as quietly as possible, being aware that what you think is quiet may still be very noisy to the person.

R

- REASONABLE: be reasonable and approach every situation with the understanding that the person is not experiencing the environment in the same way as you and adapt within reason to any requests regarding how you care for them.
- REMEMBER: when you learn something new about the illness or the best way for you to approach caring, try to remember it for another occasion.

- RESPECT: respect any requests the person may ask of you regarding perfumes, chemicals, movement, motion, noise, light and instructions.
- RESPONSIBILITY: take responsibility for your actions. Allow the person to be responsible for their choices. Be responsible in how you behave near and around the person and in their environment.
- RESPOND: respond appropriately and immediately to any request for help. Waiting may mean you lose the moment, delaying your help may result in deterioration.

S

- SILENTLY: you may find yourself in a very silent household where the slightest noise can hurt. Learn to feel comfortable in silence.
- SKILLED: you need to develop your skills and become sensitive to things that you might not have noticed ordinarily.
- SWIFTLY: respond as swiftly as is possible and safe to ensure the need is met. There may only be a tiny window of opportunity.

T

- THOUGHTFUL: a thoughtful, aware approach enables growth and empowers you in your work.
- TRYING: try your very best at all times. This is particularly important because the person's health is very vulnerable to deterioration and they are depending on you to get it right.

U

- UNCONDITIONALLY VALUE and respect the person.
- USEFUL: aim to be aware of any correct, useful information, for example helpful aids and tips on how to approach a given task.

V

- VALUES: it is important to establish your underlying values and beliefs in regard to how to care for someone with ME. Values affect attitudes and actions.
- VALUING: a valuing approach to the person will be mutually beneficial.
- VULNERABILITY: the person is very vulnerable and may be very physically frail and sensitive. You need to be aware of this vulnerability and act caringly and responsibly at all times, to develop a trusting strong relationship that is mutually valuable and flows.

W

- WITH CARE: act with care. Take care and pride in everything you do.

X

- 'X-RAY EYES': you need to be able to see all the invisible hurdles that a person with Severe ME faces in order to achieve the most basic of actions. You also need to be able to see how you can either increase the number of hurdles in any process or work to enable a smoother process for the person, to avoid worsening their experience of you and risking jeopardising the interaction.

Y

- Yes: saying yes is a healthy way to approach care. Know why you say yes to caring.

Z

- Zealous: be zealous and enthusiastic in your caring role but always apply gentleness and sensitivity to the tasks you perform, due to the physical reality of the person you are helping.

64

A WISH FOR CARERS

∼

May you keep going, when you feel like despairing, when there seems no hope of a clear way forward.

May you dare to stand up against any system or organisation that tries to deny or bury the truth.

May you find the confidence to speak up and keep speaking up.

May you look beyond the dreadful suffering to see the person, so they maintain their integrity and self identity.

May you learn to grow and learn, in spite of the suffering.

May you stay and care when everyone else leaves.

May you keep believing in love and goodness.

May you find new hopes and dreams in a reality so stark that there couldn't possibly be any, always hoping for better times for us all.

SELF-REFLECTIVE QUESTIONS FOR HOME CARERS

THE ISSUES FACING HOME CARERS are far more complex than for professional, paid carers, who should have clear boundaries, responsibilities, training and support.

When you live with a person and care for them full time, you not only have the responsibilities of caring and meeting their physical care needs, you have the complexity of personal relationship and the sometimes complicated dynamics of interacting that arises because of the nature of who you both are as people. Your expectations of each other and your learned habits also impact.

Caring changes the whole way you live together, particularly when caring is long-term it brings many challenges to overcome.

Issues facing parents might change, particularly over time, as the child becomes a teenager and then a young or older adult and the concepts of adult independence and changing relationship dynamics arise, impacted by severe illness and the need to still offer care. There is also the very real concern of what happens as you age and caring becomes more of a struggle or an impossibility.

Issues facing adults in a partnership or friendship will also include the dynamics of that relationship which may impact how you approach caring.

For children or siblings offering care or simply living with someone in the home who has Severe ME there must surely be a host of complex emotional and practical issues, that would not arise were it not for ME impacting every level of life.

QUESTIONS YOU MIGHT ASK yourself in order to better understand the complex dynamics that might ensue:

1. ARE YOU TAKING ANY OR ENOUGH SPACE FOR YOURSELF?

If so, how are you using it?

It is not necessarily enough to take space for yourself. It is how you use the time. You may need rest. You may need to do some special activity. You may want time to be creative or you may want to reflect on yourself and develop your awareness and personal growth, for example. It is important to really look at how you use your time to ensure it brings balance and a sense of right perspective to your life.

Do you need to affirm all the good that you do?

Can you think of better or other ways to be together that are not just about care, but about relationship?

2. WHAT IS YOUR PERSONAL ATTITUDE TOWARDS YOUR CARING ROLE?

Is it something that you feel good about?

Is it something that you feel obliged to do?

Does it feel that there is too much expectation and responsibility?

Your personal attitude may impact the way you feel about yourself, the person or the way you actually provide care. Do you need to own any disquiet, disappointment, frustration or change your perspective?

3. What are your personal losses?

There are many, many losses for both the Home Carer and the person who is severely disabled by ME. The grief can be incapacitating. It can also be ignored and denied within the daily demands of coping and managing daily life. When major losses occur like a death in the family or a close friend, the impact can be devastating and yet the invisibility of your existence can mean much needed support, recognition and understanding is absent or minimal. Take time to honour your bereavement processes or they may interfere with your ability to be present and care fully.

Do you have any emotional support to deal with the losses?

How can you take time to safely own and express how you feel?

4. What are the gains of caring?

There are many gains to caring. Sometimes it is easy to forget them. It might help to remind yourself, especially if you are feeling worn down or overloaded.

You may find you need to take time to nurture yourself more, if that is possible.

Take a moment each day to look around and notice the good things in your life.

. . .

5. How is your self-image affected by your experience as a carer?

If you feel you can never get it right or you overly take on responsibility for making things better beyond what is realistic or possible, you may end up feeing useless, helpless, hopeless or guilty that you are not doing enough or getting it right. At the end of the day, as long as you understand and aim to meet the care needs of the person as best you can, you still need to respect the reality that however good a carer you are, the person you love will still be suffering from the illness and the challenges you face will be the same each day because of, not because of you.

6. How many different roles are you juggling at the same time?

Multiple roles may make you feel overloaded or overwhelmed in your capacity to offer care. You may need to consider how your roles are balanced and whether they need to change or if you can safely let go of any of them. They may also affirm and bring a sense of balance and validation to you.

7. Do you feel supported and respected by other professionals who you have to engage with?

There is a very real danger that the Carer who supports and stands up for the person they care for, will end up being clientised, criticised, wrongly judged or not equally respected, especially if Professionals are recommending unsafe psychosocial therapies or simply being patronising or thinking they know best.

It is wise to remember that Professionals have a job to do,

they are not there to be your friend.

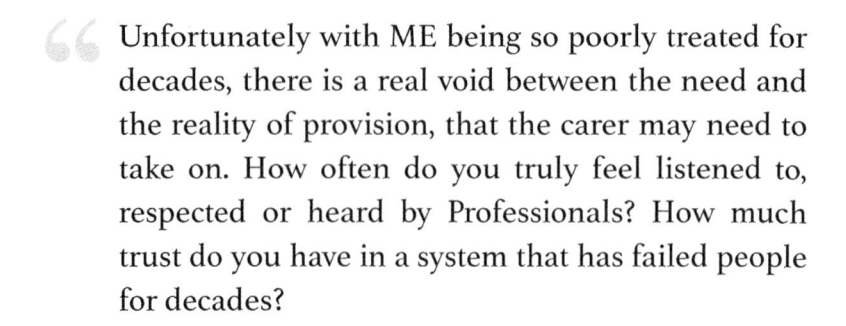

> Unfortunately with ME being so poorly treated for decades, there is a real void between the need and the reality of provision, that the carer may need to take on. How often do you truly feel listened to, respected or heard by Professionals? How much trust do you have in a system that has failed people for decades?

8. Do you feel valued for what you do?

It may not be easy to feel valued or appreciated by the person you care for because of the nature of the symptoms that they experience and how they impact every aspect of caring, making it hard to express.

You may need to look at things differently to see how important you are to the person.

9. Are there areas where you can grow in awareness?

It can help to review for yourself how you are offering care and whether it can be improved by developing greater awareness either of yourself, the environment or the other persons needs or experience. It is not necessarily easy but it may help you grow in understanding, especially if caring is a challenge due to the complicated nature of symptoms or hypersensitivities and the intense demands that they can have upon you.

. . .

10. Do you need extra support?

You may need it, but it may not be available, reliable or good enough. Nevertheless it may be possible that you can at least support each other or acknowledge need and look at new ways to meet it.

11. What sort of support would be helpful as opposed to what might be available?

Make a list.

12. What might help improve your relationship... with yourself? With the person?

It may be worth reflecting upon this to see clearly if there are areas that might be improved.

13. What do you need?

Be honest with yourself about your needs.

14. Are you feeling overly responsible for things beyond your control?

Again, be honest. It might help you see how to feel less stressed.

15. Are you seeing all the good that you do and all the things you do get right?

If not, then definitely make time to reflect and own this. It is very important to achieve balance and feel affirmed.

. . .

16. **What are the good things about your relationship and your life that you can celebrate.**

    Make a long list.

PART FOUR: COMMUNICATION ISSUES

Here we consider how to communicate in the face of multiple difficulties in understanding, thought, information retrieval and processing, articulation and two-way interaction. Many of the taken-for-granted ways of communication, for the ordinary person, do not apply for the person with Severe or Very Severe ME. Once again, we will emphasise the crucial importance of your personal posture and your willingness and ability to really listen.

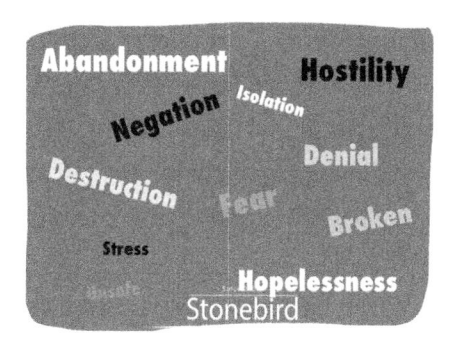

*Attitudes, values, posture and role, are particularly important.
To not feel listened to is totally invalidating.*

COMMUNICATION: A COMPLEX ISSUE

∽

EVERYONE NEEDS TO COMMUNICATE in order to get their needs met, whether it is asking a question, relaying information, interacting with others for work or other business or building relationship, for pleasure and personal fulfilment.

How easy, then, you might think, to say what you mean and mean what you say.

Yet even in the ordinary world understanding and meaning can be unclear, confused and not as straight forward as you might hope, depending on how well you articulate your information, as well as how closely the person is listening to what you are saying and also how they interpret what has been said or conveyed.

Feelings too can be hard to identify and difficult to express.

When a person seeks to communicate with someone who

has been diagnosed with Severe or Very Severe ME, communication difficulties are greatly increased.

For the person, disabled by Severe or Very Severe ME, there are likely to be multiple and variable breaks to communication.

Complex symptoms and system dysfunctions interact to cause breaks in:

- understanding
- speech
- retrieval of information
- co-ordination
- articulation
- thought
- processing of information
- two-way interaction

...resulting in an inability to type, explain, think, remember, speak when needed, use the phone, hold an implement to write, read or comprehend incoming information.

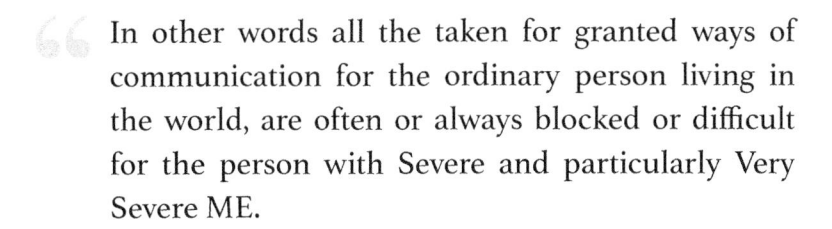

> In other words all the taken for granted ways of communication for the ordinary person living in the world, are often or always blocked or difficult for the person with Severe and particularly Very Severe ME.

This makes meeting every day need, let alone bigger needs, extremely challenging or impossibly painful and hard to achieve.

The most important lesson you can learn, perhaps, is that you cannot make any assumptions, but must watch for clues as to how the person is experiencing your presence and what difficulties they might be having in telling you their need.

You must truly listen and focus on their message.

Just because you have said something, that you think is specific and clear, does not necessarily mean that it is as clear as you think it is or has been understood.

There may also be issues with language, where what you might mean may differ from the person's understanding. This all adds up to a potential break down in communication and smooth interaction.

If you are not aware or prepared to pay attention to the fine process of communication, you may find yourself feeling any of the following:

- dismay
- annoyance
- frustration
- confusion
- feeling of inadequacy
- feeling of helplessness
- doubt
- upset

We have learned that patience and a proactive response are the best way to adapt.

Ultimately you need to figure out how:

- you will communicate
- the best times
- the best way
- what not to do or say to increase the difficulty in communication

It requires a high degree of skill, intention, perseverance, empathy, concentration, a willingness to change, alongside a critical understanding of how you interpret information and communicate yourself. How good are you at listening?

How good are you at following instructions to the letter?

For the person the effort of communicating with someone else can be extremely difficult and deteriorative, especially if they cannot flow with or adapt to their very limited energy. Severe pain, cognitive dysfunction, physical weakness or outright paralysis, noise, light, movement sensitivity or other sensitivities impose barriers upon the potential success or failure of any interaction.

It is not easy.

If a system of communication is not figured out, particularly for those who cannot speak, open their eyes or tolerate noise or light, life becomes even more painful and frustrating. The person helping or just being with the person may need to wait, if the moment is wrong, but must also understand what to do of necessity when communication is impossible. This is complex.

It takes a huge amount of time and effort to create the understanding, the routine and the precise interaction required so that misunderstanding and neglect do not ensue.

If sign language needs developing or interpreting, it may take time to comprehend the meaning.

If speech is extremely weak or quiet or very slow or distorted by paralysed lips, then the person listening must focus patiently on following the sounds and understanding what is being said. This really is extremely skilled.

Being able to observe body language and non-verbal cues is also important.

> If no communication is possible this needs comprehending by both. The effort to force it can be catastrophic.

This is why we advocate a partnership approach and a posture of openness. The reward, hopefully, is a successful two-way flow, a meeting of need in the least stressful way and a much greater sense of connection.

BLOCKS TO INTERACTION

∽

INTERACTION AND COMMUNICATION ARE not easy, straightforward or as simple as one might hope, with a person diagnosed with Severe or Very Severe ME. There are many blocks created by the illness experience itself, causing difficulty processing or understanding language, making speaking and retrieving memory and information extremely difficult to impossible at times.

However the person wanting to connect may also bring their own blocks to the relationship:

FEAR

There are many levels of fear and different ways it manifests:

- Fear of failure.
- Fear of knowing how to interact.
- Fear of not knowing what to say.

- Fear of disability or illness.
- Fear of getting it wrong.
- Fear of silence.
- Fear of feeling inadequate in the face of suffering.
- Fear of feeling helpless to help.

OPINION

This may be a direct or indirect opinion:

- Your own uninformed opinion.
- The wrong opinion of others.
- A wrong opinion gained from misinformation concerning the nature of ME and its treatment.

LACK OF AWARENESS

This can be on many levels. There may be a lack of awareness of:

- How you move, act, think, speak, relate to another.
- The other person's needs.
- The symptom impact and affect.
- How to communicate with a person with complex symptom experience and multi-system dysfunction.
- How to act around a person with severe hypersensitivities to noise, vibration, touch, light, movement, chemicals, perfumes, severe pain and extreme weakness.

INSENSITIVITY

This may be general or specific:

- Insensitivity to environmental noise.

- Insensitivity to subtle changes in energy.
- Insensitivity to perfumed products in the environment.
- Insensitivity to other people's needs.
- Insensitivity to your own needs.
- Insensitivity to non-verbal clues.
- Insensitivity to brightness of light.
- Insensitivity to the impact of your own normal actions, movements, gesticulations.

If you cannot reach out sensitively, empathically or recognise when there is a problem in the environment because you cannot notice it so easily yourself, then you may not be able to notice if there is an issue for the other person:

- You may not notice how the person is coping with or tolerating your presence.
- You may not notice if the person is struggling with the conversation or whether if what you are saying or doing is worsening things.

Hopefully this awareness will develop, over time, with willingness and an intention to develop better ways of interacting and connecting.

Thinking you know best

Each person's experience is unique and must be respected and recognised as such, in order to interact safely. Anyone thinking they know better or best, may get it very wrong if they do not listen to the person themselves and take guidance from the other person.

Lack of understanding

Without understanding, you will struggle to relate and communicate effectively or at all with the person.

There may be:

- A lack of understanding of the impact of your presence in the room.
- A lack of understanding how to effectively and safely communicate.
- A lack of understanding when to communicate, when to wait, when it is ok to carry on talking, when to listen.
- A lack of understanding of your direct impact upon the person.
- A lack of understanding that how you are, affects the interaction.

VOICE

The impact of your voice can sadly be devastating, especially if the person has noise and/or vibration sensitivity. It can be a huge block to relationship. The impact may be variable. All the following can have an affect, perhaps due to noise and vibration sensitivity of the person or the energy required to listen or the level of pain experienced or difficulty understanding or processing information or something else:

- Your voice tone.
- Your voice timbre.
- Your voices loudness.
- Your speed of speech.
- Your length of time speaking in one go or altogether.

All have an impact, as can the content of your speech and

the complexity of information, that can mean a person may not even be able to understand you or may get confused or deteriorate from contact, becoming unable then to tolerate your presence in the room.

DIFFICULTY IN LISTENING TO ANOTHER

If you cannot engage with two way interaction comfortably and far prefer to be the person talking or sharing information or stories about yourself, you may have difficulty reaching out to hear and allow the other person to express themselves or share their painful or different experience.

You may not have learned listening skills that will help you better interact. Or you may be preoccupied with your own worries and issues. You may be unaware of this until confronted with this situation.

EXPECTATIONS

If you expect the person to engage with you or be interested in the same way that they were before they were ill, you may be disappointed. The following can be a huge block:

- Expecting the person to look and behave the same as before they were ill.
- Expecting the person to tolerate the environment, the same as you do, without understanding any hypersensitivities that may alter the way the person experiences you or the environment.
- Expecting the person to follow your train of thought.
- Expecting the person to understand information.
- Expecting the person to laugh and smile. This may not be physically possible.
- Expecting the person to be able to easily listen to you or converse.
- Expecting the person to chat to you.

- Expecting the person to be able to easily repeat something, two or more times.

Expectation may need to be adjusted, especially if relatively new to this situation or if it is the first time you interact. Hopefully this will improve connection and relationship, allowing empathy and understanding to grow and develop.

69

WHEN YOU ARE FEARFUL

∽

As Dr Nigel Speight (2020) [1]comments, in the face of Severe ME the doctor might panic, leading to avoidance and neglect. I know, from my own experience of Caring, how overwhelming the stark reality of Very Severe ME can be. It can trigger all kinds of emotions, not least fear that you just do not know what to do to help.

When you are fearful, it may help to remember that:

- Fear can diminish you, through terrified thoughts and exaggerated beliefs.
- Fear can be overwhelming and incapacitating.
- Fear can block true sight and clear direction.
- Fear can alienate you from feeling compassion.
- Fear can misdirect you or lead you to inaction or wrong action.
- Fear is not the truth.

- Fear can lead you away not towards someone.
- Fear distracts.
- Fear makes you feel unsafe.
- Fear may tell you false stories.

Let fear not blind you to truth. Let fear not block you from empathy. Let fear not overwhelm you. Let fear not inhibit you from right action. Let fear not persecute you. Let fear not torment you. Let fear not misguide you. Let fear not mislead you.

∼

May fear reduce for you.
May hope strengthen you.
May truth live in you.
May wisdom guide you.
May discernment encourage you.
May inner peace fill your days.

---

1. Dr Nigel Speight (2020) **Severe ME in Children** https://www.mdpi.com/2227-9032/8/3/211/htm

70

ACTIVE LISTENING

∼

WHY IS IT SO IMPORTANT TO be seen and heard? Living in total isolation and separation can leave you feeling unconsidered, less than real, invisible, uncared for, unrecognised, unknown, belittled, less than human even. The need to be seen for who you are and what you have experienced and heard is massive.

To actively listen means:

- to give your fullest attention to the other.
- to watch for non-verbal cues as well as the words someone is speaking.
- to convey both by your posture and look, that you really care what the other person is saying.

> Even if you do not speak a word, you can still convey empathy for the person and what they are

sharing, even if that content is painful, unresolvable or distressing.

This requires awareness of your:

- posture
- body-language; how you convey yourself non-verbally

Sometimes words, opinions, positive thinking, finding solutions, suggesting actions, will get in the way of just being present and hearing the person, feeling their pain, conveying you are listening, not judging them.

Sometimes there are no answers, no solutions, no clear ways forward, just the speaking, the feeling, the sharing may be more than enough for the person. To truly be listened to and heard is fundamentally validating.

To feel safe enough to speak of a deep hurt or unmet need is everything. To have someone else's pure attention can be life bringing, affirming, healing.

To speak what might have felt unspeakable, in total safety, may be an incredible, brave first step to find balance and clarity. To express out loud and hear yourself, in a safe space, may help you to work out for yourself what is needed, without any intervention from another.

To feel affirmed, valid, valuable enough to be truly heard, can work miracles of healing or become the first step in a long process of dealing with pain, grief, deep wounds, isolation, separation.

Being affirmed makes such a difference when you live in an invisible, tormented world that no one understands or seems to care about or even notice.

71

SUCCESSFUL LISTENING

∼

WHAT IS THE DIFFERENCE BETWEEN being listened to and not?
You absolutely know, you feel it in your guts, when someone has not listened to or heard what you have actually been saying.

To be heard brings a sense of rightness, of flow, of acceptance, of peace, relief even.

An inner certainty arises from the connection made, when you feel truly that the person has listened fully to you, comprehended your meaning and heard what you have said, even if what you are saying is uncomfortable, challenging or difficult to relate to.

> To listen, really listen, is a very special gift to give another person.

The opposite can be extremely hurtful or dismissive. Not listening shuts down communication and breaks any connection that might have been possible.

It leaves the speaker feeling bewildered, shunned, shut out, discounted, disregarded, disrespected, isolated, even unsafe. At worst it is demolishing and utterly alienating.

The skill of listening is extremely important, but one that not everyone necessarily pays enough attention to or knows how to do well or at all.......

So what does it feel like not to be listened to by the different people in your life, when you are facing chronic long term illness?

MEDICALLY

To not be listened to runs the risk of your illness not being correctly diagnosed.

It can lead to your health issues being misinterpreted.

It can result in misinformation to important others.

It can make you unsafe if you are then given the wrong medicine, wrong treatment recommendation, wrong advice.

It can leave you feeling isolated, dismissed, misinterpreted, disbelieved, patronised, disrespected, hurt, helpless, neglected, harmed and more ill.

PROFESSIONALLY

Professionals have a responsibility to offer a service. How well they offer that service may, in part, be down to how well they can communicate and especially how well they can listen to their client in order to genuinely meet their need.

Attitudes, values, posture and role, are particularly

important here. To not feel listened to by a Professional is totally invalidating.

FAMILY

Family dynamics can be complex and can easily get in the way of being listened to or heard. The interactions and patterns of communication may be very set and rigid, not necessarily open to growth or allowing someone to be seen in a new light.

This may depend in part on the relationships and the power held by different family members and the level people generally relate on.

> Not everyone can do 'deep' listening and genuine sharing. Attitudes and values can make a huge difference as to whether you will feel seen or overlooked, tolerated or cared for in a conditional or unconditional way.

Health, being busy, work demands, poverty, worries, stress or other responsibilities or interests of individual members, may also influence their availability to listen. Roles and personalities also can be very set and hard to break out of or be enabled to change.

Concern may be genuinely felt, but not easily, if ever expressed.

Sadly, without a willingness to be open and listen, an intention to hear and respond, to convey genuine interest and caring for the other, misunderstanding can arise and relationships can become shallow, blocked, disharmonious or absent and almost permanently broken or lost.

. . .

FRIENDS

When you need a friend to listen to you, especially when the dynamics of the relationship have changed, you may or may not find the compassionate listener that you hope for. It really depends on the nature and parameters of the friendship in the first place; how mature or aware the person is and how much they want or are able to really reach out and hear you in your need.

The topic or content of what you want to say, may not be of interest, of enough concern or the person may just not be capable of hearing or dealing with any deeper emotions or complex issues that you might want to share. If illness, injustice or grief are present, loss and bereavement may also come between you, especially if you no longer can be or do what you used to be or do.

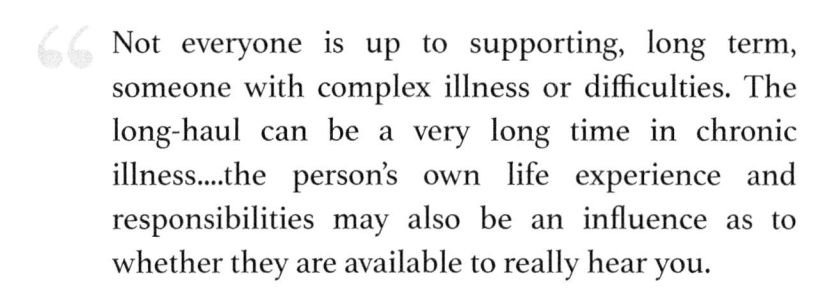

> Not everyone is up to supporting, long term, someone with complex illness or difficulties. The long-haul can be a very long time in chronic illness....the person's own life experience and responsibilities may also be an influence as to whether they are available to really hear you.

PARTNER

The break in communication that can come between partners, when one does not feel heard and seen by the other, can be extremely painful. This is especially so, if loss and grief are involved, for the stages of grief can bring overwhelming, unexpected, painful denial, anger or sadness to the surface.

It can be helpful to try and put any disappointment or

negative experience in context. Though this is not always easy or necessarily possible, especially when you are feeling very ill.|

It might help to consider:

What might underlie the failure to connect and communicate?

What has led to the experience of not listening?

- Is it wrong timing?
- Is it unrealistic expectation?
- Is it overwhelming need?
- Is it the way you have expressed yourself?
- Have you misjudged the other person's ability to listen and hear?
- Are you both unwell or in pain?
- Is it because your lives and abilities are so different from each others now?

It could be a range of issues. It might simply be that the person does not have enough time to listen accurately or attentively, they may be too busy or distracted for a range of reasons to pay attention. They may have something they feel is more important or interesting to think about. Perhaps they feel out of touch because of the impact of the illness?

They may not be able to tolerate, comprehend or emotionally deal with any emotional or factual content you need or want to share.

∼

A NEW APPROACH TO LISTENING

. . .

LISTENING IS a skill that can be developed and progressed, but it requires commitment.

Compassion, interest, concern, genuineness, equality, open heart and mind and the desire for true connection, lie at the heart of good communication.

Sadly not everyone might experience or know this.

> It may even, for some, be deliberate disinterest or false judgement, based on prejudice or wrong assumption, that blocks listening.

This is much worse than the person who genuinely is unaware of their lack of ability to listen and hear.

It may be down to a lack of capacity to empathise or simply an inability to easily convey to you that you have been heard. Or the person may simply not want to listen too much, which can be painful to know.

There are other possibilities to consider though; for some, there may be a lack of valuing or comprehending the importance of listening. If you have never been fully listened to yourself or felt the need to be really heard, you may not know how to do it or how important it is or what a difference it can make to your relationship.

There are no easy answers, to broken communication and feeling disregarded and unheard, but the starting point could be to attempt better two-way communication, trying to understand the others position and reactions. This might be hard or challenging or impractical or too difficult to manage, depending on who it is, their role and relationship to you and how ill you might be.

> But perhaps if you can understand context, at least it is a starting point to not feeling demolished, when you do not feel that you have been heard, especially by someone you care about.

This can be important both from the Carer perspective, if the Carer does not feel seen, heard, appreciated or listened to by their ill partner, by their family, by the professionals that they have to engage with.

It can also be equally true for the ill person. They have the additional symptoms that block communication and being together, being able to listen, comprehend communication at all or even minimally.

Successful listening entails a range of skills.

SKILLS AND REQUIREMENTS OF LISTENING:

The following are some things that might help to develop a proactive listening relationship:

- Enough time
- Patience
- No distractions
- A safe space
- Attentiveness
- Honesty
- Open heart
- Compassion
- Empathy
- Ability to concentrate
- Reflecting back what you have heard accurately
- Ability to pay close attention to emotional content

- Genuine interest and concern
- Ability to focus on the other person
- Willingness to engage on difficult subjects
- Acceptance of how the other person is feeling
- Hope of understanding
- Respectful engagement
- Ability to hear without judgement, excuses or blame
- Unconditional valuing of yourself and the other person
- Ability to accept expression of emotion
- Understanding how to communicate and what impositions might be placed on communication by the illness

It make take time and a commitment to develop a good listening relationship where both feel heard and respected. This is the fundamental concept behind a **Partnership Approach to Caring.**

> A person living with a very severely disabled person with Severe or Very Severe ME will have to adapt to and accommodate the complex impact of the symptoms themselves, while trying to listen.

They are a huge barrier to two way communication.

Listening then may need to focus very much on limited language and non-verbal communication and it may take longer to arrive at understanding.

72
HOW TO LISTEN TO EACH OTHER

∼

Down many years of intense, indescribable suffering, trying to connect through every conceivable level of broken interaction, this is what we have learned:

- Listening, really listening, means your heart is open, your ears are alert and your eyes are really seeing the other.
- There are no words necessary.
- There is no separation, just pure awareness flowing between you.
- Here you see, here you hear, here you know; all in a moment of wonder and connection that no words can describe.
- This is the truth of listening.
- This is the true of feeling listened to.

- This is the truth of being heard.
- Everything is held in a pure moment of being, all is understood.
- All is touched, felt, healed and made whole.
- All is absolutely well between you and the person, even though nothing may be well anywhere else.

73

HOW YOU MIGHT APPROACH COMMUNICATION WITH SOMEONE UNABLE TO DIRECTLY SPEAK TO YOU

∼

THIS SHOULD BE APPROACHED with care and sensitivity. It requires awareness, a person-centred focus and great commitment to get it right.

If you are going to speak to the person, you need to think about your tone of voice, pacing of words, content and loudness. These can make all the difference between comprehension and a complete obliteration of meaning.

For someone with processing difficulties, who may not be able to understand or follow conversation, the wrong way of communicating can add to the sense of isolation, separation and any potential inner turmoil.

If you speak slowly, using the minimum amount of words, there might be more chance of the person following and at least getting the gist of anything you want to say, assuming they can tolerate the sound of your voice at all.

You may have to consider how to indicate non-verbally that you understand or need to know something.

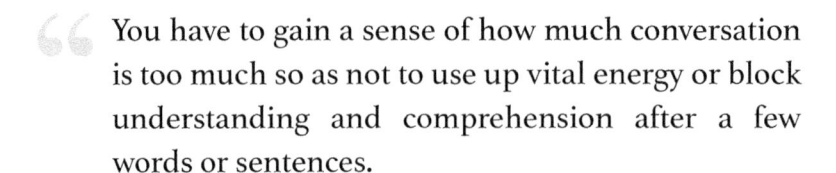

> You have to gain a sense of how much conversation is too much so as not to use up vital energy or block understanding and comprehension after a few words or sentences.

You need to look for non-verbal clues as to how the person is receiving your words. This is assuming that your voice is tolerable and that the sound will not trigger symptom deterioration or intensification of pain or use up too much energy, adding to the post-exertional overload.

It is not easy to communicate with someone when their normal pathways are broken or damaged. There may be moments when understanding is more likely and interaction may be more tolerable, though it may be unpredictable, variable or not possible.

Choosing the wrong moment to speak and expect a response can be catastrophic for the person.

You may need to think of alternative ways of communicating, for example learning the person's own unique sign language, if they have developed any.

If the person is not palsied, too weak to smile, nod or convey understanding with their eyes, learn how to read their particular facial expressions,

Passing notes, whether hand written or by text or email, if the person can deal with technology, might be a way of sharing information. But always remember the brightness of the screen or the unexpected sound of a phone ringing might be excruciating or painfully unacceptable. Perhaps there is a possibility even, of written simple two way dialogue.

Remember, though, that energy and ability may be limited.

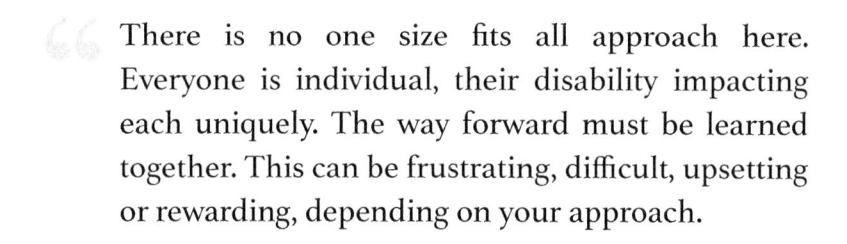

> There is no one size fits all approach here. Everyone is individual, their disability impacting each uniquely. The way forward must be learned together. This can be frustrating, difficult, upsetting or rewarding, depending on your approach.

The important thing to remember, is that no matter how broken the pathways to connection are, the person before you is still intrinsically themselves and of equal personhood. There is no excuse to patronise or diminish the person further, speaking over them, speaking at them or about them as if they are not there. Nor is treating an adult like some sort of grown-up child or object or precious doll, acceptable or valuing.

You have to learn how to keep respecting the person and their space, their needs, their personhood and equality.

You need to look for ways that the person, who cannot speak, may be trying to convey something to you; they may, for instance, make certain sounds, point with their eyes or head. It is really important to be open to seeing communication as two way.

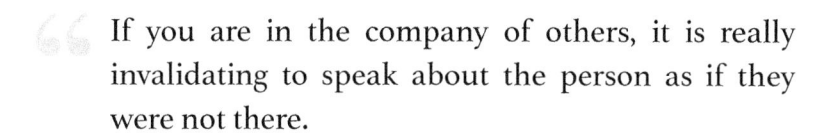

> If you are in the company of others, it is really invalidating to speak about the person as if they were not there.

Try to develop inclusive ways of speaking with, for and to the person. Never assume that they do not understand if you speak in their presence about them and for them. Also make sure you understand that even if the person's language is limited, they still need to feel respected and valid. You can still have meaningful, two-way interaction, it just needs to be more sensitive, aware, perhaps slower, with enough space to allow any possible response.

How You Might Approach Communication

- Listen to what the person might be trying to say.
- Look for any signs of communication.
- Observe non-verbal responses and posture.
- Convey warmth and interest.
- Talk inclusively at the appropriate time.
- Affirm the person.
- Give feedback on any conversation that you might have had on their behalf.
- Speak directly to them.
- Let them know that you are present and listening.
- Be aware of how their symptoms will be affecting their ability to tolerate your presence.
- Show respect for them and also for their environment.
- Be reassuring.
- You may need to explain things in advance of doing them to ensure an inclusive approach, taking symptom experience and timing into account.
- Find patience.
- Be centred, be willing to engage with the person in the best way for them to feel included and seen.

PART FIVE: IMPACT UPON RELATIONSHIPS

Here we look at the profound impact of Severe and Very Severe ME, upon relationships.

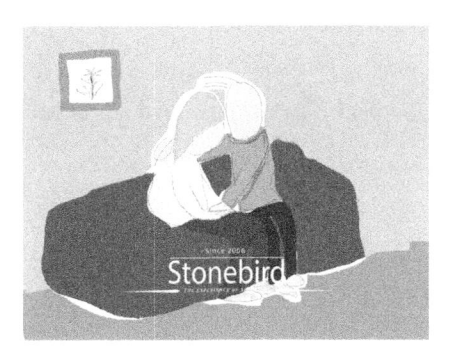

When very severe chronic illness invades your world it brings a profound encounter with your own limits, paradox and mystery.

INTRODUCTION TO VERSES FROM INVISIBLE OCTOPUS POEM BY CORINA DUYN

I am honoured that Corina Duyn has not only shared an extract from her latest work here, but also one of her fabulous images to accompany it.

Her poem powerfully highlights the devastation of the illness experience, which is so out of anyone's control. In a beautiful way Corina expresses and shares her own journey and how she finds solace in nature and particularly birds.

VERSES FROM INVISIBLE OCTOPUS
POEM BY CORINA DUYN

∼

The reality of life
with the unpronounceable illness
Myalgic Encephalomyelitis
is hidden and fragile

ME as Invisible Octopus
acting as puppeteer
keeping me upright
or stumbling at will

inflicting pain
challenging my brain
its crushing weight
taking my breath away

I live in a disbelieving world
my reality
trivialised
dismissed

https://www.corinaduyn.com/site/poem/

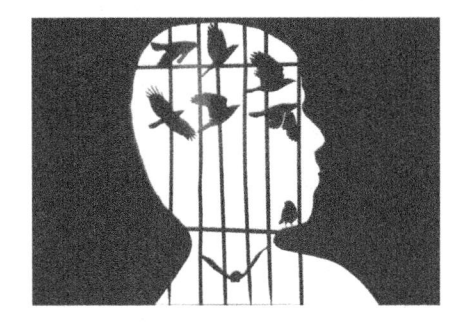

77

A MOMENT IN TIME

∼

YOU NEED TO GRASP THIS idea that a moment in time can make all the difference to the person with Severe and Very Severe ME; that even when something is totally impossible in one moment, it may be achievable in the next. We daily hope for better moments.

Often it may seem as if there is an empty space around the person, in which nothing is possible, yet if you are paying enough attention and are willing, able, gentle and patient enough, there may be a moment in which you can achieve something together.

78

ON BEING A PARTNER TO SOMEONE WITH VERY SEVERE CHRONIC ILLNESS

∽

FOR ANY RELATIONSHIP, THERE is inevitably, over time, a challenge to grow, to deal with change, to face adversity together.

When very severe chronic illness invades your world, however, it brings a profound encounter with your own limits, paradox and mystery. You are daily confronted on multiple levels with loss and grief alongside a need to rise above it all and find your true self, still shining, even in the deepest chasms of pain.

The immense physical, emotional and spiritual stresses and strains of a situation where the other is long-term ill and disabled can trigger anger, despair, a sense of hopelessness and helplessness. It is so important to aim to keep stress for you both to a minimum, if possible. Stress complicates everything! It may mean fundamentally changing your life and the way you interact. It is not easy but it may be necessary in order to achieve some balance, rest and a way forward.

[1]**You must look after yourself well.**

In the face of the seemingly overwhelming needs of the profoundly ill person, it is possible to overlook your own needs as well as not see or understand the other's experience and recognise what they need and how to provide it. Both people are equally important, yet may have very different needs and ways of meeting them. The task becomes, long-term, how to do this in a mutually loving and respectful way. Inevitably this is difficult at times, the path may not always be simple, clear or easy to follow.

When difficulties occur, it is particularly important to take time when possible, to be still, to reflect, to process what has happened, what you have learned, what you have experienced and felt. To look at what might be missing, to see things differently, to find a new way of doing things.

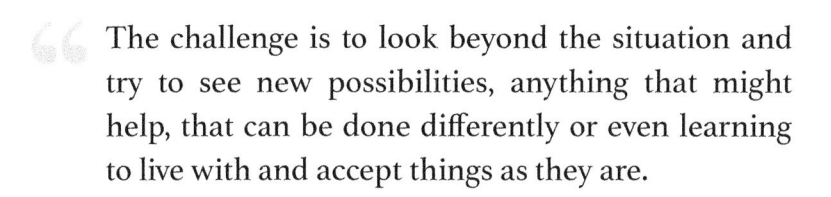

> The challenge is to look beyond the situation and try to see new possibilities, anything that might help, that can be done differently or even learning to live with and accept things as they are.

Sometimes a personal journal helps for learning and reflection, an acknowledgment of disappointments, of hopes and of personal feelings, even those more difficult to speak about or express. I have kept a journal for many years. Over that time, I have grown immeasurably as a man and learned better how to express myself and articulate issues and feelings. I have grown to accept that I am far from perfect, with a gathering tranquillity and sense of peace, liberation, joy even, but never complacency!

I have learned the importance of doing things that you really like to do, even if they need adapting for environmental reasons, in order to do them, such as composing music only with headphones on.

It is important to find things that you can enjoy and can bring happiness, fulfilment, fun, peace, uplift and renew you, without feeling guilty perhaps. For me that is gardening, cycling, web design, playing and writing music. These all uplift me; yet I have had to develop careful ways of doing them in order to not negatively impact my wife, who is profoundly noise sensitive.

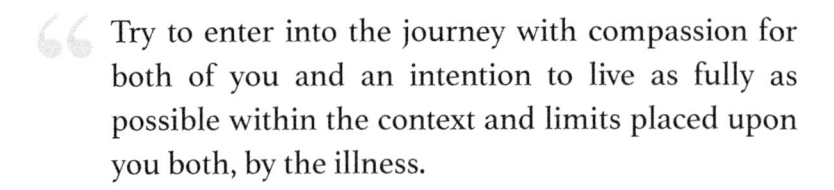

> Try to enter into the journey with compassion for both of you and an intention to live as fully as possible within the context and limits placed upon you both, by the illness.

The way forward is not always clear, straightforward or easily achievable. I can only speak for myself, but I have known a balance between joy, in its simplest, purest form, alongside sorrow, in some very bleak places indeed.

Often I have had to dig very deep, to find some chink of hope, in the desperate times. Yet, still, I have been privileged to know a depth of love, closeness and connection that touches an equally deep mystery. I am so grateful for that. Be kind and generous to yourself. Aim to acknowledge what is brave, good, noble, amazing about you. That is so important. Learn how to be loving to yourself, if you have not learned it already.

Recognise all the good you do.

Try to maintain your own identity, never let it get totally swallowed up into the role of being a "Carer" or the intensity of suffering. You have many aspects to yourself. Nurture them all, when you can. Caring always starts with caring for yourself. Only then are you in a strong position to be with someone so ill, so in need of your strength and presence, but don't forget it is a two-way relationship and the other person still has much to offer with love themselves, despite the illness.

You can ultimately only do this together.

---

1. In Severe/ Very Severe ME, the illness constantly shifts in its barbarity, you have to be acutely aware, there is no room for even a moment's complacency.

   The slightest things I do, in all innocence, can so easily be devastating to my beloved, my clumsy attempts to help can have the most appalling consequences, my presence can be too much to bear at times.

   Truly the most ill, in their depths of suffering, are trapped in an unimaginably terrible, lonely place of relentless torture, crushing hypersensitivity, paralysis and agony.

   Sometimes, when things are very, very bad, no contact whatsoever with the person is possible.

   I find that the most difficult challenge of all, especially when my actions are the trigger.

79

YOU FIND A WAY

WHEN YOUR WIFE'S LIFE is torn apart by Very Severe ME you care, you seek answers, you speak up, you do your own research, you find a way to muddle through

You find a way to help her.

You see her being harmed by ignorance.

You see her disappearing from the world.

You see her struggling to bear the unbearable, with no pain relief whatsoever and an intolerance to drugs.

You see the illness not just take her body from you, but her mind badly affected, her sight diminished, her creativity trapped inside, her talent unexpressed, the possibility of motherhood lost for her; her tears tear at you.

You hold out a hand if she can bear to tolerate your presence or your contact - so often not possible.

SEVERE AND VERY SEVERE ME: THE UNEXPECTED LOSSES

∽

WHEN YOU SUDDENLY COLLAPSE, disappear from your normal life and are labelled with a diagnosis of Myalgic Encephalomyelitis, aka "ME/CFS", you unexpectedly enter a no-mans land. Nothing is as it was before. Everything is impacted upon, either subtly or wholesale. An "ME/CFS" diagnosis is far too vague to accurately recognise or identify the underlying physiological disorder that underpins your devastating inability to think or move.

ME/CFS is a vague conglomerate term, that covers up a range of disparate illnesses that are viewed as fatigue conditions, rather than the WHO neurological disease that the name Myalgic Encephalomyelitis originally represented, when first coined and was associated with enterovirus. Because the ME/CFS label you have been given is non-specific, without clearly identified physiological congruence and a safe, specified, appropriate biomedical treatment pathway, you may not be given the same medical respect of any other recognised physical disease.

Your losses have already begun to multiply. The complex losses you are faced with, not only from the consequences of the devastating, disabling, life changing illness you are experiencing, but also more insidiously from the ambiguity of the medical profession towards it and their lack of knowledge of how to safely help you, means that fundamentally your person, your self-image, your integrity, your rights, your truth, can become fundamentally assaulted too.

You are thrown into a completely unfair, unjust, unsafe situation. The provision that you might expect from falling ill in general, does not seem to apply to you once you have been given an "ME/CFS" diagnosis.

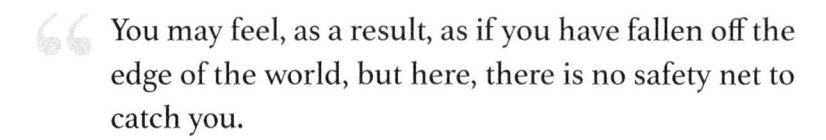

> You may feel, as a result, as if you have fallen off the edge of the world, but here, there is no safety net to catch you.

Anyone else, diagnosed with a long term, disabling or terminal disease, will most likely have some sort of medical support, general recognition, medical knowledge and understanding, a treatment pathway based on pathology or at least long term support and follow up, kindness and empathy for their situation, though we recognise that for rare diseases or particular circumstances, this may not always be the case.

Into the secret, hidden world of a person diagnosed with Severe or Very Severe ME, then, may come completely unimagined, unexpected, multi-level losses, that can hit you all at once and sadly never stop coming.

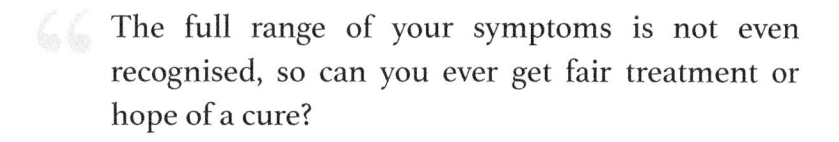

> The full range of your symptoms is not even recognised, so can you ever get fair treatment or hope of a cure?

- Misunderstanding
- Misinterpretation
- Mistreatment
- Misrepresentation

are rife in ME world, negatively impacting your whole life potentially.

Here are some of the losses that you may experience:

EXTERNAL LOSSES

- The loss of confidence in the medical establishment
- The loss of respect for many professionals
- The loss of security and trust in the systems meant to protect the vulnerable and disabled
- The loss of confidence in the diagnosis you have been given
- The loss of respect for many of the 'experts in the field'
- The loss of expectation and hope to be seen, heard, validated, helped and accurately interpreted
- The loss of trust that you will be fully medically investigated by those in positions of power and responsibility
- The loss of belief in systems and people who fail you again and again

- The loss of provision of an accurate and reliable diagnosis and treatment protocol
- The loss of trust in politicians and charities who say they speak for your disease, then misrepresent it
- The loss of trust that doctors will follow the spirit of the Hippocratic Oath and first and foremost, 'do no harm'
- A loss of trust in the integrity of 'ME' research

ENVIRONMENTAL LOSSES

- A loss of being able to go where you want, when you want
- A loss of tolerance of every day things
- A loss of being able to block out sound
- A loss of being able to engage with other people, reliably, safely, repeatedly, predictably or at all
- A loss of tolerating speed, motion or movement near or past you
- A loss of mobility within your external and internal environment
- A loss of every normal thing that you had come to accept as the norm
- A loss of tolerance of perfumed products and people who wear or use them
- A loss of free, easy, simple interaction, whether in person, by phone, by writing etc
- A loss of tolerating ordinary light

PERSONAL LOSSES

- Loss of career
- Loss of family contact
- Loss of income
- Loss of health
- Loss of wellbeing
- Loss of independence
- Loss of ability to communicate
- Loss of tolerance
- Loss of 'being yourself'
- Loss of feeling
- Loss of sensation
- Loss of security
- Loss of memory
- Loss of control
- Loss of proprioception
- Loss of movement
- Loss of energy
- Loss of muscle function
- Loss of creative ability
- Loss of friendships
- Loss of public celebrations
- Loss of figure
- Loss of self-image
- Loss of respect
- Loss of roles
- Loss of family contact
- Loss of enjoying ordinary every day things
- Loss of intimacy
- Loss of physical tolerance for contact
- Loss of vision

- Loss of speech
- Loss of food tolerance
- Loss of pleasure
- Loss of sensation
- Loss of comprehension
- Loss of understanding
- Loss of words and language
- Loss of expression
- Loss of presence in the world
- Loss of presence in your family
- Loss of connection with others
- Loss of social interaction
- Loss of faith
- Loss of hope
- Loss of action
- Loss of activity
- Loss of peace
- Loss of spontaneity
- Loss of dignity
- Loss of identity
- Loss of interaction
- Loss of time
- Loss of hopes and dreams

INTERNAL LOSSES

- A loss of connection between mind and body
- A loss of connection between thought and action
- A loss of connection between intent and actuality
- A loss of connection between hope and possibility

- A loss of connection between eye and hand
- A loss of connection between desire and ability
- A loss of connection between thought and mouth
- A loss of connection between action and memory
- A loss of connection between need for rest and being able to rest
- A loss of connection between reading words and comprehension
- A loss of connection between need and being able to get the need met

THE POVERTY OF SEVERE AND VERY SEVERE ME

∼

THE POVERTY ENTERED INTO here is a stark and complete poverty. It is a poverty on all levels:

POVERTY OF WEALTH: unable to earn money you rely on benefits which are not easily gained or easily kept, neither do they provide for more than the minimum of life.

POVERTY OF PRIDE: you have to sacrifice all self-esteem as you search more and more for charitable grants to meet your basic needs, crushed by rising prices and dwindling funds

POVERTY OF FAMILY: you become alienated from their normal lives, they shut you out, they get on with normality rather than enter into the path of suffering with you, that you endure moment by moment, too careless of your feelings, too busy in their own lives, too angry with you for not being who they want and expect you to be.

POVERTY OF NEIGHBOUR: you are unable to maintain contact, reciprocate favours, join in social events; you become isolated even from those in closest proximity.

POVERTY OF FRIENDSHIP: people simply get fed up with your lack of presence, with the difficulties of communication, they cannot and do not understand, nor do they necessarily want to be that flexible. You become less visible, they move on and forget you, you become at best a Christmas card or birthday card, more easy to maintain than any genuine relationship that has emotional costs and complexities involved.

POVERTY OF LOCAL COMMUNITY: you are not seen or heard, not being able to engage on their terms, you become invisible, yet you also feel judged for it.

POVERTY OF RELIGION: the religious who cannot reach out beyond a general 'do good, feel good' factor that meets no real need. They do not visit or genuinely reach out to connect. Church becomes an impossibility to attend. Prayer groups become an impossibility to attend. Interaction dwindles away to nothing, if it was ever possible. People walk past on the other side of the road. There are no 'good Samaritans' here it seems; not in the long term anyway, in our experience.

POVERTY OF SOCIAL NORMS: you simply cannot comply with normal expectations, meetings, deadlines, red tape, procedures, social gatherings, social events, any external demand.

POVERTY OF UNDERSTANDING: many people simply do not understand the vast complexity of need nor the physical suffering a chronically ill person experiences; they are often thought of or represented as people who have made themselves ill, due to wrong thought and laziness, considered scroungers on the welfare state, a waste of space, completely denied access to help, without huge battles to get even their basic needs and rights met.

POVERTY OF KINDNESS: there is a shocking ignorance in the general public, even in those closer to a person, diagnosed with Severe or Very Severe ME, that leads to unkindness, thoughtless gestures, ablism, exclusion, hurtful comments and all because of ignorance and lack of a genuine desire to enter into this place of pain and stand by you in this very difficult, often bleak place. Few bother, few dare to care enough, others are thoughtless or deliberately unkind and uncaring.

HERE WE LIVE, ON THE EDGE OF SOCIETY, ON THE EDGE OF HEATH CARE PROVISION. ON THE EDGE OF SURVIVING.

SEVEN USEFUL HABITS TO DEVELOP WHEN YOU LIVE WITH SOMEONE DIAGNOSED WITH SEVERE/VERY SEVERE ME

WHEN YOU LIVE WITH AND choose to offer care and support to someone in great need, that care must be of a high calibre and convey a high level of sensitivity to the person and how their symptoms manifest.

It greatly helps if you can develop certain habits that will create a strong basis from which to proceed.

These seven habits, if you choose to develop and sustain them, can help strengthen your role in a way that brings confidence to yourself and reassurance to the other.

They can help you flow in your relationship and your necessary role as care-giver, even in difficult situations, where you need to respond effectively, efficiently and certainly.

1 CREATE AN AWARENESS WITHIN YOURSELF, OF YOUR ROLE

Develop an awareness of the role and expectations of the role. Are you there as a partner or in some other family role, or are you providing a specific care role or a combination of both?

If you have to perform a specific caring task, learn to keep your mind and attention focussed on that task in hand, so that your own personal situation and interests do not distract you from doing your very best.

Learn to see the boundary around your role as carer, what delineates it, what is required for it? This may not be so clear when you are a home carer. It might help if you have a clear picture of the care you need to provide within the context of the wider relationship role that you have with the person.

For example, preparing a meal for yourself and your partner is something anyone might do in relationship, preparing a meal for someone with food intolerance, needing a highly specific diet, needing to eat at specific times in specific ways in silence, due to noise sensitivity and then helping the person eat it, will require a care-centred approach where specific care needs, the how, when and what must be done, are an additional focus. But never forget the relationship aspect, the partnership approach to caring.

Someone who is noise, light, touch, movement sensitive deserves your very best attention in order to not get harmed by the slightest wrong sound, flash of light, gesticulation, pressure. This is not easy, especially when living full time with the person, however, if you can create a habit of being extra careful always, around the person or in the home, it can become become a habit, that can make your caring role easier and more natural to you and more effective and rewarding for you both.

This may not come naturally. You may need to adapt the way you do things in your wider life if you live in the same space as the person you care for, so that both your needs are met and your relationship is sustained and strengthened.

. . .

2 Develop empathy and understanding in your practice

In order to help someone in severe pain with multiple sensitivities and little to no energy available to speak or move it helps if you have a level of empathy and an understanding, to the best of your ability, of what they might be experiencing and how you might impact upon them. This will take time to develop, it may not come naturally at first.

Listening and reflection are key elements. If you do not understand the way the person experiences contact, sound, movement, chemicals and perfume, light or your presence in the room, it will be more difficult to offer support and help in the right way.

If you can learn to read the signs, you may be able to determine if it is safe to talk, to ask a question, to proceed with necessary contact. This can become a conscious habit. Look for the level of pain upon the person's face. See how shallow or weak their breathing is. Notice if they are flinching, just by you moving gently in the room.

Learn to adjust your pace to their need. Learning to wait for the right moment is a huge skill. Gaining understanding as to why this is so important and more than that, essential, is to develop empathy for the person you care for, which can only enhance your interactions.

3 Get in the gentle flow of living and caring

There are many actions and reactions in yourself that you take for granted, such as numerous gesticulations you might make whilst explaining or talking enthusiastically about something, moving quickly, busying about your day, loudly opening cupboards or chopping food up, singing out loud to yourself, for example, that would cause pain and deterioration in the person you care for, if not checked, in their presence. They are not wrong of themselves, but may be too much for the person you care for to cope with.

Again, this takes massive effort on your part, to restrain your natural tendencies in order to flow more calmly, gently, caringly with the person. You need to learn the best way to flow with the person in order to help them and make your own life easier at the same time.

> A sudden hand gesture might cause confusion, shock, disorientation, irritation or deterioration. yet it is only too natural to gesticulate without thought or awareness.

Talking too loudly and enthusiastically might be overwhelming, too much information to process, too painful to hear, too difficult to follow and understand. This can be upsetting or disappointing if you have things you want to share but the person cannot understand or process what you are saying.

Moving quickly might completely sap their energy, overload their senses, cause noise inadvertently, confuse the person with slow processing ability. But moving slowly needs conscious effort if it is not your natural style. Banging cupboards might cause shock or muscle weakening, intensified pain or headache, even paralysis in someone with profound noise sensitivity. A little extra care can make such a difference.

The sound of cutting up food might trigger ear or head pain, muscle spasms, irritation. Ways to manage achieving specific tasks need to be developed and habitual to save time, effort and help avoid deterioration. None of this is likely to be normal to you. It has to be learned in order to flow better with the person, whose health can literally depend on the quality of care and the way you generally are around them. The attention you place on how carefully you provide help or the way you generally interact and flow with the person can makes all the difference, probably more than you realise.

4 BE MORE CONGRUENT WITH YOUR VALUES AND ATTITUDES: 'WALK YOUR TALK'

It is helpful to recognise what your values and attitudes are towards caring. For example, the Stonebird ultimate value is enshrined in our motto:

'...you don't have to do anything to be of beauty and value in the world. Even if you cannot move, even if you cannot communicate, even if you cannot think, still you are precious and your presence matters.' To live this value is to believe in your own intrinsic goodness, both from the point of view of carer and person needing care. And whilst we believe it with all our hearts, yet still we may struggle to feel it at times, when the illness gets intolerably hard to deal with.

To offer support to the most severely ill, you need to be flowing as congruently as possible with the person and yourself.

It is one thing to say you have a certain value or attitude, it is much harder, in practice, especially when faced with complex situations with no easy solutions, to both maintain your value base and respond congruently within it; walking your talk as opposed to saying you have a value base, but not living by it. In our experience this is a deepening and a rewarding process over time.

The more you look at your practice and the way you live, paying attention to how you might flow more congruently from your values and beliefs, hopefully with kindness towards yourself and an openness to look and grow more harmoniously, the more hope there is of integrating your beliefs and values into your life and flowing together as a natural habit.

5 DEVELOP A FLEXIBLE AND ADAPTIVE APPROACH TO NEED.

One might think of habit as being inflexible, rigid, stuck. However, a habit can be positive as well as limiting or negative. A learned, positive, proactive habit will hopefully mean that your automatic response is grounded in a helpful confidence that you are certain of yourself. This is especially important when faced with a crisis, when you need to respond calmly, sensibly and proactively.

You cannot be too rigid in these circumstances. You need to develop an open, caring, responsible approach that enables you to meet each need tenderly in the right moment in the best way, with agreement from the other.

6 CARE FOR YOURSELF AS WELL AS CARING FOR OTHERS

This is not such an easy habit to develop. It is easy to get the balance wrong in either direction, either being too focussed on self or too selfless to look after yourself well. In order to care well and safely, however, you need to be able to pay attention to your own needs, so that they do not invade the space required whilst providing particular, specific care needs for someone else. Only you can know what your needs are. Only you know how you can allocate time to meet them. This is a delicate balance and may need negotiating, one that is a helpful habit of getting into.

. . .

7 Be open to new ways and possibilities

It is important to know what works and what does not work, when you live and care for an extremely ill, hypersensitive, vulnerable person, with multi-system dysfunction and unexpected reactions. These things that work safely and well, should be learned into known, reliable habit for best effect. However, when you need to work out new ways of doing things together, you might also need to be open to doing things differently.

To achieve this you need to be able to see the issue clearly facing you and to be willing and able to think around the situation to figure out possible new ways of achieving the help required. Safety, security and risk assessment must always be factored in to any action.

In our own experience, there has had to be greater focus on how to interact and what can be done safely and when.

A commitment is required to really want to make life better or an understanding that in order to do this, I, not the person, may have to change, in order to try to make things more tolerable and maximise the quality of our interactions and being together.

Be careful then of what habits you develop. Make sure, if you can, that they are habits that enhance both your lives!

LEARNING TO LIVE IN SMALLER SPACES

This was a piece written before our Silver Anniversary.

∼

I FIND AGEING WITH CHRONIC illness to be a very strange experience, especially when that chronic illness is diagnosed as the much maligned, misunderstood, misinterpreted Myalgic Encephalomyelitis and when the diagnosis is Very Severe.

Large swaths of time disappear into an empty, nothing existence, where time appears to have stopped altogether, the only experience being pain and isolation from everyone and everything, even yourself, whilst at the same time, finding it has simultaneously jumped or leap-frogged over most major events, without even a smile of recognition or suitable celebration.

No contact possible, the family gatherings mount up and

fall over with neglect and you are no longer thought of or expected to participate. Visits become painfully difficult or impossible, dialogue then becomes one-sided and even that hurts and is painful or hard to follow. You have nothing to tell except excruciating agony and a disappeared life, so tiny by comparison that the normal person simply would not know how to exist within it, so small the experience, so inadequate the celebrations, when seen from worldly view.

You try to cling on to who you were, to talk as if you know about things, as the years go by and they diminish into unreality, a life once lived becomes bizarrely unrecognisable to life lived now.

So many things lost. No social life. No children. No holidays. No careers. Little money. Little status. So many hopes and dreams let go of, not possible at first, still not possible 25 years on and so you learn to adjust, to see the world differently, to hope in goodness rather than specifics. You become disconnected from the outside. You are filled from the inside, if you are filled at all.

You learn to live in smaller spaces, in new ways, you focus on the moment, for any other moment beyond now is unpredictable, unreliable, uncontrollable. And when the next moment comes, it is still mostly empty of all possibility. And yet you carry on, holding on for better moments, new ways forward, hope an elusive star that shines, at intervals, to guide you forward.

There is a deep sadness about the passing of time, that cannot be comforted away, for it is lost, even to memory, for the mind-blanking spaces of paralysis destroy everything in sight.

And so the 25 years of our marriage - which should be and still are - an amazing celebration, have to be celebrated in a totally alien way to most.

For despite the horror, the torment, the despair, the torture experienced again and again, and all that living with a Very Severe ME diagnosis throws at us, still, for us at least, there is a solidity, a continuity, a flow of love, that beats all illness, that transcends all suffering, a constancy of commitment beyond the impossible, where most would have walked away and given up with the sheer impossibility of most moments, yet we have stayed together and amazingly continued to love each other, finding meaning within our lives, forging a way forward, despite the negation, the neglect, the downright harm done by some and the almost complete dearth of medical integrity that is required yet rarely found in this particularly medically ignored disease.

And so when it comes to our Silver Wedding, we look back together, unable to share our celebration with others, unable to have a party, unable to go out to a pub or a restaurant or a cafe or to go anywhere at all, to have a special meal.

Yet we hold on to each other, on that most special of days and we find a depth of meaning in the simplest things that we have shared together - moments when we have clung on and survived the most desperate of experiences.

So many memories of beloved garden birds who have become our friends; the robins, the doves, the blue tits, the great tits and the blackbirds, who have graced our lives down many years, so many precious moments with our two much loved Corgis, one now sadly gone, greatly missed, both who have loved us and blessed us beyond imagining, awards won, videos made showing the truth of this devastating neurological disease, proud as anything of all the numerous things Greg has done for us all down the years, especially speaking up at the Gibson Inquiry in Parliament, publishing books, articles, creating websites, developing the MOMENT Approach, to try and keep people safe, always committed to truth and integrity - no small feat as an unwaged carer, caring for his tortured wife.

> *We feel proud of all the things we have had to fight for and all the times we have won.*

Our hearts shine when we look at our garden, grown from nothing, one plant at a time, over many years, when we think of the huge pleasure, from the smallest thing: seeing a ladybird snuggling in a Hollyhock bud, holding our breath while a baby robin jumped on my foot, feeling the wind in my face, easing the never-ending pain for one tiny moment, no centimetre of my body, pain-free, focusing on the pure, elegant beauty, of a single rose, opening to the bluest sky above it, waiting, then finally seeing the tiny sheaths of grass emerging as they push through the soil, growing our own lawn from scratch.

The triumph of Greg baking me a sugar-free, dairy-free, hydrolysed oil-free, amazingly delicious, gluten-free cake, a hand held, a look of love, a candle lit every year at 3pm, a prayer said; all these things are a great strength, holding me against unimaginable pain, so many intolerable moments held in love, triumphing purely because of that love.

A marriage vow stronger than iron. That indeed is something incredible to celebrate!

84

BE THE CHANGE YOU WANT TO SEE

5.30 AM, A GLIMPSE OF the rising sun, through a hedgerow, fills me with hope, for this new day. So how is it going to be? Inevitably it is going to be painful for my wife, constantly shot through with agony, paralysis, inability, profound, tortuous hypersensitivity, unbelievable torment.

BUT HOW AM I GOING TO BE WITHIN IT?

...distracted, withdrawn, irritable, tired, bored, listless, unable to bring any light to the situation, do anything much at all?

OR WILL I MAKE ALL THE DIFFERENCE TODAY?

...by being present, alive, interested, open, aware, gentle, warm, welcoming, willing to help, to think things through, work them out together?

Will I know joy, will I experience togetherness, partnership, miracles, will today be wonderful, despite the atrocious suffering, in the moments in between, even if just in glimpses, even if just for a second or two?

Here, in the beauty of dawn's first light, I know how much is down to me, to how I will choose to be today.

"Be the Change You Want To See in the world", the late, great Stephen Covey once wrote.

Isn't that the truth?

Being with Linda has taught me this, over and over again: that if I want the day to shine, I must shine. If I want the day to flow, I must flow, if I want the day to be loving, I must love, if I want to make a difference today, then I must be different.

A brand new day. All is fresh and soaked in Spring time dew and light reborn, no wonder the bird song is so tremendous.

Treasure every fleeting moment, don't waste one precious second of it, they seem to sing.

PART SIX : PROFESSIONAL INPUT

Here we look at the implications of Severe and particularly Very Severe ME for professional care givers.

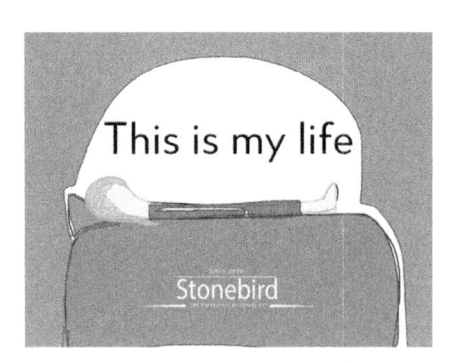

It is a massive risk for anyone diagnosed with Severe or Very Severe ME to let any professional into their life.

INTRODUCTION TO "DOOR POSTER" BY SOPH CLARK

I am delighted that Soph Clark has given me permission to share the Door Poster that she uses to warn people of her hypersensitivities and how they need to be, in her presence.

It is a brilliant example of some of the information professionals and visitors need to know before they enter a room or try to engage with someone with Severe or Very Severe ME.

Each person will have their own instructions on how to approach them safely, which may vary slightly from this example.

A DOOR POSTER BY SOPH CLARK

∼

Hypersensitivities:
Light / Sound / Touch / Motion Vibration / Smells!
Please READ Before Entering!!!
Disinfect hands before entering!
Please whisper! You will HARM if you don't!
Door stays closed at all times!
One person talks at a time!
Keep speech simple & slow!
No loud noises! eg. paper / phones!
No banging / bumping of bed / floor!
Don't put anything on the bed! Including yourself!
No fast / sudden movements!
No bright lights! eg. phones!
No harsh smells! eg. perfume!
Keep a respectful distance from me!
Do not hover / stand over me!

Do not pressure me to do anything I say I cannot do!
NO means NO! Don't ask me again!
Family member has permission to talk on my behalf!
Do NOT ramble / talk too much!
Do NOT talk until I signal it is okay!
No dog allowed!
Please be sensitive to my needs / wants! If you do not follow my rules...
You will be asked to LEAVE!
Thank you! 🙂

ORIGINAL LIST *by Soph Clark (shared with permission)*

RISK ASSESSMENT IN SEVERE AND VERY SEVERE ME

~

It is a massive risk for anyone diagnosed with Severe or Very Severe ME to let any professional into their life. Very Severe ME is particularly so outside anyone's normal experience that it is extremely hard to comprehend or understand or know how to safely engage with the person.

> Our (painful) experience, over decades, has taught us the importance of making sure that professionals behave safely. Trust has to be built not assumed.

Information, therefore, should be provided, in advance, to the person concerning the knowledge, experience, attitude and expertise the practitioner has. The person with Severe or Very Severe ME needs to know who they are about to trust potentially with their life. They need to be sure that the person really knows about Severe and Very Severe ME, how fundamentally physically ill and vulnerable people are and how to safely interact and not cause deterioration.

More than this, they need to know what the professional understands by the term "ME" and how they interpret it.

> Risk Assessment should concern not only the interventions but also the interactions. If you do not come from an organic interpretation of illness, you will not be coming from the right understanding required.

Given how every nuance of movement, speech, timing, noise exposure, light exposure, physical contact, cognitive demand, of any interaction, can be neutral, helpful or harmful, a careful consideration of how to approach the person should be included in the Risk Assessment.

The practitioner should be aware not only of what their intended intervention might be, but how they will carry it out:

- timing
- flexibility
- how they enter the room
- how they communicate with the person, based on individual need
- what clothing, colours, materials they wear
- how any movement might impact upon the person
- how perfumed products of any sort may impact
- what level of light is tolerable
- the risk of symptom deterioration

There is much to be learned about how to safely engage

with the person and how the illness impacts them, before any intervention can be safely suggested. It is essential that the practitioner's understanding of the illness and how they interpret it is made clear.

Risk Assessment in Severe and Very Severe ME requires an organic approach. Apart from awareness of the disease itself, it should be based on knowledge and awareness of how anything the professional might do, or anything they might ask the person to do, may affect symptom exacerbation or health deterioration.

The Risk Assessment should proceed from a partnership perspective in which the individual and/or their chosen representative has personal input regarding their physical experience and needs. Safety should be the primary thought.

Symptom reaction and hypersensitivities must be included in the assessment; general assumptions will not do at this level of need and severity of illness. It is too easy to get this wrong.

The person must feel safe and reassured that they are listened to, heard, acknowledged and respected, not misinterpreted or ignored. The person's environment should not be contaminated or impacted negatively by any home visit.

Any inadvertent harm by unaware practitioners or inappropriate recommendations or poor contact must be avoided.

Risk:

R= **Respect.** You must respect the person and know how seriously, physically ill they are.

I= **Intent.** Your intention, above all, must be to do no harm.

S= **Safety.** You must approach the person with massive sensitivity, taking full account of their acute environmental hypersensitivity and full symptom experience in order to safely engage with the person.

K=**Knowledge**. You must have relevant and up to date medical knowledge that safely informs your practice. You should have an idea of the impact of any suggestion or interaction and the dangers of post-exertional deterioration.

These are the key components.

Any suggested pathway or intervention must involve an explanation of any potential risk, impact or side affect, specifically in relation to Myalgic Encephalomyelitis.

A plan for what to do if deterioration occurs, following engagement, needs to be in place and responsibility taken. It is important to ensure that the person has fully comprehended the information and the intention.

A person should never be left harmed, deteriorated, their life made impossibly difficult to manage, from a home visit, through a lack of awareness or knowledge. Video appointments rather than outpatient's appointments should be routinely offered for those too ill to engage or go to hospital. GP's should be willing to do home visits when required, though these might be a challenge or too hard to directly engage with.

Personal accountability and accuracy of recording information are essential.

How you approach and perform a Risk Assessment with such severely physically disabled people, needs careful consideration in order not to trigger deterioration. The right way to engage must be sought. The avoidance of health deterioration is an absolute.

Information must be presented simply. This may mean that a representative advocates for the person or enables communication.

Any Assessment, whether conducted face-to-face or remotely or by some other means, should be agreed to be a fair and correct representation by both the professional and the person or their representative. Any written information provided by the person should be fully respected.

Any forms provided to the person, must be kept confidential and worded appropriately, with enough space to write answers in.

It is utterly traumatic to trust a professional to come into your home and your life only to find that they have written reports with information that they have literally made up, which they will not change and which misinforms others and misrepresents you. Once a professional has let you down, wrongly assessed you or inaccurately recorded you, it can have a lasting impact.

There is no excuse for it.

REASONS WHY IT IS INAPPROPRIATE TO OFFER COGNITIVE BEHAVIOUR THERAPY TO SOMEONE DIAGNOSED WITH SEVERE OR VERY SEVERE ME

We cannot comprehend how anyone would think it would be appropriate to offer Cognitive Behaviour Therapy (CBT) to a person diagnosed with Severe ME or Very Severe ME. However, if CBT is suggested the following concerns are important to note.

How can someone with variable ability to think, speak, process, understand, find answers and retrieve information, possibly tolerate or engage with the CBT process, ever?

A Risk Assessment would surely raise awareness, or highlight the following potential issues:

- The complex environmental issues that may block the practitioner even being in the room with the person.
- The physical difficulties accessing normal communication media such as a phone, computer, tablet.
- The complex severe cognitive issues and post-

exertional deterioration that accompanies mental or physical effort in Severe and Very Severe ME.
- The danger of ignoring or denying or not comprehending the impact of how questions affect the person. The use of energy for mental processing may mean energy for physically dealing with other needs may be reduced or impacted negatively. Asking tediously obvious questions or irrelevant questions, emotively loaded, may waste precious energy resources and mental function.
- The broken communication channels that limit and impact interaction.
- The great danger of misinterpreting symptoms and making any wrong assumptions about their cause.
- The post-exertional impact from using your mind, trying to access parts of the brain that do not work well or only sporadically.
- The risk of over-stimulating adrenalin, which has a negative impact on the body and gives the false impression of better health than is true.
- The danger of setting unrealistic goals and pushing the person into worsening cognitive dysfunction and symptom deterioration/exacerbation.
- The variability of memory, both to find answers specific to the assessment procedure and the ongoing ability to remember instructions and alter thoughts.
- An inability either long term or sporadically to access or process thoughts.
- The difficulty in retrieving information.
- The sheer impossibility of actually answering questions as part of the process and therapy.

- The difficulty of poor memory impacting the ability to remember what you are supposed to think in order to help yourself change your thoughts.
- The difficulty of dealing with any emotional experience or situation, due to severe lack of energy and ability.
- The risk of being misunderstood, misinterpreted or wrongly labelled with a mental health condition.
- The inability to follow goal setting strategies due to the nature of the diseases and severity of symptoms and the symptom backlash during or after interaction.
- The difficulty of learning anything new or even retaining what is already known.
- The risk of harm just engaging with someone let alone actively trying to change or improve a situation.
- The fact that even if someone can engage once with another person, it does not mean that this is repeatable or predictable or safe.
- The inappropriateness and danger of setting and linking goals to activity increase in any form or by any name.

One would hope that a Risk Assessment would be comprehensive, rigorous, insightful and that it would be made by aware, objective, open-minded practitioners who understand the physical nature and reality of Severe and Very Severe ME. A general tick-box list would be unlikely to record the detail needed.

Any assessment needs to be done with awareness, sensitively, carefully and appropriately.

It should highlight the complexity and potential dangers of any interaction, let alone something as cognitively challenging as CBT.

The person being assessed needs to agree any assessment.

There is a danger of professionals:

- Not fully recording responses
- Misinterpreting responses
- Not asking the right questions
- Not listening to the answers
- Being too impatient to wait
- Not having enough time to give to the process
- Not accurately recording what has taken place
- Literally claiming the person has said or agreed something that they did not

This must be avoided.

On top of these issues are the very real problems and challenges, particularly people with Very Severe ME face, regarding interaction of any kind for even a moment, let alone a therapy session.

Some of the difficulties that come to mind are:

- The danger of mental or physical overstimulation.
- The barriers imposed by sound sensitivity, light sensitivity, movement sensitivity, perfume sensitivity.
- The difficulty of tolerating someone in the same room.
- The difficulty of not having enough energy or physical ability to engage with someone else.
- The inability to have two-way conversation.

- The inability to process and understand what is being asked.
- The severe to profound level of symptom experience a person may be experiencing.
- The inability of the person to manage should their symptoms be inadvertently worsened, short or long term.
- The very real likelihood that the information/conversation will be forgotten, due to severe cognitive dysfunction.
- The great vulnerability of being misinterpreted, mislabelled as mentally ill or misunderstood.

We conducted Severe ME two patient surveys,[1] one which showed that only 4% of participants found CBT helpful while 96% found that CBT had a negative impact on them.

---

1. It is striking how much the experience of the severely affected is comprehensively ignored. In conjunction with the 25% Group, Stonebird conducted a regional and national surveys of people with Severe ME, to try to affect change locally for a biomedical service in Norfolk and nationally for the Gibson Inquiry. This publication is an attempt to rectify the situation. The voices in these documents are of immense importance; their experience of ME is infinitely more extreme than the mainstream, many of whom may not have Myalgic Encephalomyelitis in the first place. These surveys reflect an almost total lack of understanding of this marginalised group. It is to the NHS's shame that people diagnosed with Severe and Very Severe ME still receive little to no service or support.
   https://stonebird.co.uk/psurvey.pdf

THE CORE COMPONENTS OF A PROPER ME SERVICE

For 27 years and counting, we have lived in hope that the NHS would provide a safe, appropriate medical service for people diagnosed with Myalgic Encephalomyelitis (ME), a complex multisystemic disorder, involving profound dysregulation of the central nervous system immune system dysfunction, cardiovascular abnormalities and autonomic nervous system dysfunction.

Despite numerous engagements at both local and national level, there is still no such service available.

This is not an exhaustive list, just some suggestions, that we would still like to see come about.

- A specific ring-fenced definition of what "Myalgic Encephalomyelitis" means, incorporating the historical truth of its association with Enterovirus and Polio[1]. Without it a service is unsafe and its client group unidentifiable.
- A Separation of "ME"[2] from "CFS"[3]. ME is a specific

disease, CFS [4] is a syndrome of symptoms, sometimes used to mean ME, other terms incorporating a wider group of poorly recognised or undiagnosed conditions and meaning a much wider group of people. This ambiguity leads to confusion.

- Complete redundancy of the term "ME/CFS" and "CFS/ME"[5]. This is a conglomerate term, it has no place in defining or recognising the neurological disease Myalgic Encephalomyelitis. The term helps no one get right treatment or recognition, it continues to promote the wider definition of fatigue illnesses under the umbrella term and often has the adjunct "aka Myalgic Encephalomyelitis " attached to it incorrectly. No one is safely or clearly identified under this umbrella label.
- Correct diagnosis to ascertain who has ME and separate other conditions, alongside the use of better criteria to define ME, for example the International Consensus Criteria (ICC), although this could still be improved upon.
- [6] A specific category of "Very Severe ME"[7] needs to better identified, with clearly identifiable criteria. This profoundly ill, severely disabled, fragile group needs to be recognised as such, in order to be better protected, rather than incorporated into a broader category of "Severe ME", which accommodates a much wider group of ability and needs. Only 2% of people have Very Severe ME.
- [8] The categories of ME to include a Symptom Severity Scale for each symptom, in order to build up a better picture of disability. The term "Severe ME "is usually associated with being bed bound,

however it does not indicate the reason for this state of being. We advocate better acknowledgment and recognition of individual symptom severity to provide clearer understanding of the experience. Not everyone would be totally bed bound in this category, yet could still be very severely disabled and have a diagnosis of Very Severe ME.

- Honouring the full symptom experience of ME alongside a relevant severity scale.
- A full biomedical approach provided by practitioners highly trained in working with people with "ME", not "ME/CFS", or any Psychosocial model of interpretation.
- A commitment to better recognise, investigate if necessary, treat if possible and support all symptoms, including paralysis. Typically many symptoms go unrecognised or under described and people are left to get on with them to the best of their ability.
- Appropriate care and support for the the acute hypersensitivities people experience. The hypersensitivities found in Severe and Very Severe ME are not well recognised, explained or supported.
- Ensuring accountability and responsibility through conducting proper, accurately recorded, sensitive, aware medical Risk Assessments. It is extremely challenging to learn how to safely be with someone with Severe and Very Severe ME without triggering deterioration, even long term harm.
- A flexible, moment by moment, not a rigid approach to care, provided by practitioners fully aware that

ME is a neurological disease, not a mental health condition.
- The provision of a medical help line, specifically for ME and emergency support for those in need.
- A person-centred, partnership focussed approach to providing care, taking into account the person's complex communication issues and severe symptom experience.
- Appropriate guidance on how to approach and individually help the most ill in a way that will not cause harm or trigger deterioration or place unnecessary or inappropriate demands upon them.
- Person-centred, Individual Care Plans appropriate for the level of severity of disability and symptom experience, recognising that the most ill will be unlikely to have enough energy to engage with people or get their basic needs met without risk of deterioration or severe symptoms exacerbation, if they can engage at all. It is important to listen to what the person needs and work it out how to meet the need safely. We would not expect the Individual Care Plan to be goal-orientated, rather we would hope it would be realistic, quality-of-life and care-orientated and flexibly provided.
- Complete recognition of how inappropriate it is to set goals and tasks for a person with Severe or Very Severe ME to achieve, rather a Care Plan should be about how to avoid deterioration and how to offer practical, quality of life enhancing support.
- The removal of "Rehabilitation" as a primary intervention in Severe and Very Severe ME.
- Biomedical home visits by Consultants and from all

fields of medicine, as necessary, for those unable to leave home or travel. Some people, however, may not be able to tolerate even home visits or face to face contact, especially without very careful preparation, understanding, flexibility and awareness. They must not be wrongly judged, misinterpreted as refusing health input. Health support must be appropriate to need and work around the person's reality and risk of deterioration.

- The provision of appropriate aids and equipment, especially for the most ill. People with Severe and Very Severe ME desperately need disease specific aids and equipment developing. This would be a new area of expertise.
- All Doctors and Nurses to be trained in a biomedical interpretation and understanding of the disease. Great care has to be taken in choice of Training Provider, to ensure they have the correct values, attitudes and knowledge and experience. Unless all doctors are taught correctly that ME is a WHO [9]classified disease involving profound dysregulation of the central nervous system (CNS), immune system dysfunction, cardiovascular abnormalities, autonomic nervous system dysfunction and provided with correct up to date information, there will continue to be a poor level of recognition, understanding and appropriate interventions and support on offer.
- A commitment to ensure that no psychiatric misinterpretation of ME is possible.
- A global willingness to think outside the box and find new ways to reach out and enable

consultations, testing, investigations and desperately needed services for those unable to access them safely or at all, for example through a mobile ME Clinic.

---

1. Nancy Blake (2016) has written an excellent history: **Lost In Translation – The Me-Polio Connection And The Dangers Of Exercise** https://www.prohealth.com/library/lost-in-translation-the-me-polio-connection-and-the-dangers-of-exercise-14079

    Dr Byron Hyde (2020) explores in depth how ME and Polio both affect the same brain areas. Please see https://docs.wixstatic.com/ugd/5b307e_06f1c3f9d3bb41539f9fde712e739c8b.pdf

2. In 1956, Dr. A. Melvin Ramsay had formally coined the name "benign myalgic encephalomyelitis", to describe the 1955 Royal Free epidemic which affected 197 nurses, doctors and ancillary staff. (Acheson 1959)

    At that time it was understood that ME, a "paralytic illness of world wide distribution " (Acheson 1959):

    Follows a contagious epidemic and endemic infectious disease.

    Represents a diffuse Central Nervous and in some cases a Peripheral Nervous System Injury.

    Can be devastatingly painful.

    Is an illness that follows an infection, probably viral in nature.

    Is most commonly seen in (a) health care workers, (b) children and older students in residential schools, nurses residences and hospitals, (c) in military barracks.

    Has definite evidence of paralysis occuring in 50- 80 per cent of patients. (cf. Acheson 1959)

    Ref: Acheson E.D.(1959) **The Clinical Syndrome Variously Called Benign Myalgic En-cephalomyelitis, Iceland Disease and Epidemic Neuromyasthenia**

3. The term 'chronic fatigue' was not associated with this illness at all, until after the name was changed from ME to Chronic Fatigue Syndrome (CFS) in 1988 in the US.

4. Although they are used synonymously unfortunately ME and CFS are not equivalent terms. ME is a neurological disease, CFS is a made-up term that encompasses a wide range of fatigue conditions.

    • CFS includes Chronic Fatigue, a mental illness, many undiagnosed conditions such as Lyme and other poorly diagnosed illnesses and undiagnosed rare diseases, as well as some people with ME, a neurological disease. Others with neurological ME may unfortunately be wrongly diagnosed as having functional somatic disorder; it is therefore unsafe,

unreliable and unrealistic to equate CFS with ME, given they are identified by different criteria.
- Currently some people use the term synonymously to mean both are mental health conditions, some interpret it as neurological; doctors and health and social service practitioners can chose which interpretation they use. This is unacceptable and dangerous for all.
- ME does not exist on a continuum with Chronic Fatigue or CFS any more than Cancer, or Multiple Sclerosis does.
- ME is not a fatigue illness, in the way it is contextualised in CFS; you don't even have to have fatigue to have ME. ME is identified by its unique post exertional autoimmune response and post exertional fatigue, which is quite different from ordinary fatigue - particularly the way it responds deleteriously to exercise.
- A service cannot safely identify and aim to treat ME patients whilst also using the CFS definition, which inevitably includes people with other conditions as well, without doing a gross disservice to patients.
- The ICC criteria for ME are very specific, whereas the criteria for CFS are far too vague, undefined, unreliable, too broad to be of any practical value.
- The International Consensus Criteria (ICC) is very clear that 'fatigue syndrome' or 'chronic fatigue syndrome' are not to be conflated with ME.
- The WHO have repeatedly clarified that diseases cannot be encoded under more than one rubric. The term CFS covers many different conditions, which may or may not include ME.
- The techniques used in the therapeutic treatment of Chronic Fatigue are not just inappropriate but potentially damaging, dangerous, even life threatening to someone with ME.
- Because of the imposition of the CFS label upon their disease, people with ME are seriously deprived of proper medical tests, treatments and research. This is cruel and unacceptable, wrecking lives, leaving numerous patients suffering for decades with no hope of a cure or treatment.

All the time there is a focus on general fatigue people with ME will continue to be negated and harmed.

5. The literature is complicated by the use of different terms, such as CFS, CFS/ME, ME/CFS or CF (Chronic Fatigue), all meaning different things to different people. Even if a person uses the word "ME", it is not necessarily referring to the original disease Myalgic Encephalomyelitis, for it depends on which definition they choose to recognise.

   "CFS" is not a single diagnostic entity and "fatigue" is not a disorder, it is a symptom; a non-specific label which embraces many different medical and psychiatric conditions in which tiredness and fatigue are prominent.

6. The International Consensus Criteria (ICC) For ME (2011) uses the original clinical term of "Myalgic Encephalomyelitis", in stark contrast to the prevailing vague, fatigue-based "ME/CFS".

The ICC provides a framework for the diagnosis of ME that is consistent with the patterns of pathophysiological dysfunction emerging from published research findings and clinical experience. (Carruthers et al 2011)

To be diagnosed as having ME :

A patient has to meet the criteria for: **Postexertional neuroimmune exhaustion**

They also have to have at least one symptom from three of four neurological impairment categories :

Neurocognitive impairments
Pain
Sleep disturbance
Neurosensory, perceptual and motor disturbances

At least one symptom is required from three **immune/gastrointestinal/genitourinary impairment** categories .

And at least one symptom from **energy metabolism/transport impairments** .

7. Words can have such a bland affect, they can under-describe or dismiss the true reality or severity of experience. Words can mis-label, can be omitted, can make something tormenting sound almost harmless and insipid.

    I have a diagnosis of Very Severe ME, yet how can I trust that diagnosis? Why would I want it at all, when it has left me tormented, mistreated for decades and irreparably harmed in the past, because the underlying physiology had not been adequately sought or understood?

    It explains nothing of my true symptom experience.

    In all honesty, no one, right now, is currently safe because:

    1. they truly do not know what is physically wrong with them
    2. they do not know why they are so very ill
    3. they do not know why they are still denied proper recognition.

    Saying you have ME, sadly, is still not enough to guarantee safe treatment or understanding

8. I asked on Social Media: If you look up "ME/CFS" on the internet, just about every site lists the symptoms as "Fatigue, Pain and Sleep". I wonder is that YOUR truth? There were many replies. The list of symptoms is a far cry from the diminishing term ' fatigue.' For the full list please see : https://stonebird.co.uk/FC.pdf

9. In 1969 the World Health Organisation formally classified myalgic encephalomyelitis (ME) as a neurological disorder in its International Classification of Diseases (ICD 8: approved in 1965 and published in 1969: alphabetical Code Index Volume II, page 173). For much more information I highly recommend you read **The Power of Propaganda**,(2017) by Margaret Williams http://www.margaretwilliams.me/2017/power-of-propaganda.pdf

TRAINING FOR PEOPLE WHO HAVE TO ENGAGE WITH A PERSON DIAGNOSED WITH SEVERE OR VERY SEVERE ME IN A CARING CAPACITY

High quality training, based upon values and attitudes, is at the heart of any good service for people with Severe and Very Severe ME. Practitioners may be skilled but not necessarily ME-aware. All training needs to be directly related to the disease ME specifically.

Training is crucial, currently however, it is weakened by:

• inadequate definition of ME, poor criteria and symptom recognition

• difficulty diagnosing accurately exactly what disease(s) the person has

• entrenched attitudes and values that do not understand, accept or just pay lip service to the biomedical reality of Myalgic Encephalomyelitis.

Training needs to include:

1 Information on the nature of the disease, including up to date high quality medical research and knowledge[1]. It is important that the people who know their experience best are

included in providing training and information, to check for accuracy.

2 **The teaching of correct underlying values and attitudes.** It is not safe to assume that any professional will have the correct biomedical attitudes underpinning their interactions and interventions.

SOME GENERAL POINTS THAT PRACTITIONERS NEED TO KNOW:

- How to approach and respect the person in their own environment, the interpersonal awareness required.
- What it means to be present to someone with Severe or Very Severe ME.
- That the person may have difficulty communicating their views, due to physical disability and cognitive difficulty.
- That the person with Severe or Very Severe ME is physically ill and severely disabled.
- That it is highly inappropriate to adopt any posture that is critical or even subtly judgemental.
- How to approach and interact in an open, honest, genuine way.
- That the person's experience is real, not false or mentally controllable.
- That there is unimaginable physiological breakdown going on in the person's body.
- How to approach the person recognising the fundamental importance of Environment, Impact, Communication, Safety.
- That the person may not be able to tolerate, process or understand speech fully or at all, or the information being conveyed to them.

- That the person may not be able to tolerate anyone, near them or in the room at any given time.
- How to approach the person in a caring way with enormous flexibility and patience.
- How to develop awareness of what triggers deterioration in the person.
- How to perform their professional role in an appropriate ME-aware way.
- How to create a safe and appropriate environment for those able to tolerate it.
- Any specific skills relevant and specially adapted to the person's need.
- Safe Assessment procedures and skills.
- Integrity in report writing and record keeping.

And above all, practitioners involved in any caring role, need to know how to work flexibly in the moment with people.

3. Courses need to be tailor made for each group that needs training and information. We would advocate an **experiential, interactive, self- directed approach** to learning, which enables the person to determine their own learning path and grow in confidence and direct knowledge through experience, though some may prefer a more didactic approach.

4. Training should be available for all levels of health care provision: Consultants, GP's, O.T's, Physios, Speech Therapists, Anaesthetists, Dentists, Nurses, Social Care staff, basically anyone who comes in contact with people with Severe and Very Severe ME.

Parents and family members, carers and others new to the disease might be interested in learning or gaining high quality information, but keep in mind that they are often the real experts in how to safely engage and understand the person they care for and should never be treated as an unequal partner, patronised or wrongly judged.

> The risk of harm is unquantifiable and the deterioration of severity unpredictable.

All can gain by developing specific awareness of how to safely engage with people with ME. It would tremendously help the ME Community as a whole. Particular care, however, needs to be exercised with people diagnosed with Severe or Very Severe ME. It requires great thought and preparation, for each person's reality is so complex and individual.

∼

FOR MORE INFORMATION on a Carer Self-Reflective learning programme please see my Pocketbook Course, Care For ME.

HERE IS A SHORT EXTRACT:

How Aware Are You of the Following?

1. THE IMPACT OF NOISE UPON THE PERSON YOU CARE FOR
How noisy are you doing every day chores and personal tasks? How quiet do you need to be?

. . .

2. How careful and sensitive you are to the person, as you perform any tasks required

How gentle are you? How rough might contact feel, even if you try to be gentle?

3 The timing of interactions and help

Are you able to be flexible? In what ways? What constraints do you have?

4. The impact of perfumes that you wear, including perfumed laundry liquid and products on your clothing, upon the person

Can the person tolerate them? Do they affect their health or well being? Have you thought about it? Do you need to take any action?

5. The sound and volume of your voice and the way you communicate

Do you notice if the person is straining to hear you or if they are sound sensitive and require you to whisper or communicate in some other way, wait a moment or try again at another time? Is this something you need to develop more awareness of?

---

1. Unfortunately research into ME generally has been hampered by a paucity of large, high quality, hypothesis-driven studies, and controversy around diagnosis. (Nacul et al (2020) **How Myalgic Encephalomyelitis/Chronic Fatigue Syndrome (ME/CFS) Progresses: The Natural History of ME/CFS** https://www.frontiersin.org/articles/10.3389/fneur.2020.00826/full)

DENTISTRY ISSUES

∼

DENTISTS NEED TO KNOW the best approach and how to interact.

A national, full, home-visiting Dental service needs to be on offer for the most ill who simply cannot travel to or tolerate a hospital or clinic environment.

It is so important that dentists have information about what is safe in terms of drugs, anaesthetics, amalgam etc. however it is difficult to get this all the time the underlying physiology of ME is so poorly identified and comorbid or alternative diagnoses are so difficult to gain.

> It is only when we started insisting on looking at heart issues, blood pressure shifts, oxygen levels ourselves, that we discovered that there were underlying problems, which could impact not only dental work, but any medical procedure, as well as

any other drug interventions or practical suggestions.

Within the context of Severe and Very Severe ME it is crucial that for those with extreme hypersensitivity, dentists understand the impact of

- noise
- vibration
- light
- voice
- touch
- perfume
- chemicals

It would help if they have some prior knowledge of how to approach the person safely.

It is worth considering the difficult reality of dental work for people with complex symptom experience:

How do you perform a filling, for example or provide false teeth, when:

- a person has hyperesthesia
- cannot tolerate pressure or contact
- cannot tolerate noise, nor protect themselves in the normal way with ear plugs or ear defenders, making drilling a torture
- has perfume sensitivity that renders the environment a hazard and chemical sensitivity that means the anaesthetic and chemicals used are potentially endangering to health, cannot lie back at

an angle or lie down safely, without weakening or paralysing?

And how do you deal with extractions if you cannot safely go to hospital or a dental surgery and there is no home-visiting service that can attend to it?

These are the very real issues that people face and there may be other issues too, for each individual person. So far, they have no easy or apparent answer.

> Without better medical knowledge about ME, people remain unsafe and any intervention is risky potentially, especially if the health issues facing someone, have not been identified, because it is 'only ME'.

People deserve to know better about what is physically wrong with them, so that they can see other health professionals safely, knowing that they will not have wrong treatment given them due to physiological ignorance.

Especially for very severely affected, it is important that people are protected from poor information or misunderstanding due to psychosocial misinformation, misinterpretation and mistreatment or the perception that they are choosing not to have treatment rather than that the awareness and ability required to safely provide it, is missing.

Due to the nature of Severe and Very Severe ME appointments need to be flexible. Cancellations, due to health issues that realistically will occur, must not be used as an excuse to block people from the service.

ACTING AS AN ADVOCATE

You have to stand firm for the truth of ME and the person's reality especially where others are limited, misinterpreting or compromising the need.

> The physical reality of ME is not negotiable nor open to compromise.

It is a serious neurological disease, with multi-system dysfunction that has a profound effect on the person's life.

Do not be fobbed off with something that is not suitable but makes the other feel self-justified, or makes you feel you have done your best or tried. It's not about making you feel better, it is whether the person is negated and their need goes unmet.

A Rule for an ME Advocate:

- You are responsible to represent the person, not yourself.
- You are standing in for the person, to get their needs totally met, to speak for them.
- There may be two sides to a story but you need to be clear which side you stand on; it is the person's.
- It is your duty to be assertive on behalf of the person you represent, even if it doesn't come naturally to you. Anything else will lead to the potential negation or minimising of the person's reality.
- Compromise concerning health or symptom experience is unacceptable.
- You need to be polite but you don't need to be popular; you need to be assertive for the truth however uncomfortable that makes you feel.
- You can't make everyone happy necessarily. The person you are trying to please is the person you are advocating for. Unfortunately with ME everything is compromised because the term "ME/CFS" compromises everything. Make sure you don't compromise too.
- You have to come from a centre of truth and integrity, with a lived commitment to understand the person's reality. Too much care is focused upon clientising people rather than empowering and enabling them.
- Your position is the assertion of the person's equality of person-hood.
- You have to be very clear about your boundaries and who you represent.

NOT A PATIENT FOR THE INEXPERIENCED CARER, BY WENDY BOUTILIER (GLOBAL ADVOCATES 4 ME-ICC)

> *As I detail in my free Ebook on the politics of ME, "Straightjacketed By Empty Air", we all owe a huge debt to Doctor Melvin Ramsay who in 1956 coined the name "benign myalgic encephalomyelitis".*
>
> *Wendy Boutilier's website, GAME, which promotes the work of Dr Ramsay is an essential visit, if you really want to understand the disease.*

NURSING IS A HEALTHCARE profession that involves years of training and continued specialized education to care for patients in a variety of settings. Nurses are often the first healthcare professional that patients meet. They are a technical expert, an educator, a counselor and a resource for the family, using all senses to better care for a patient.

It is vitally important that they understand the complexities and implications of Severe Myalgic Encephalomyelitis. Their knowledge of illness combined with exceptional people skills provides comfort and stability. For many patients, this relationship is an anchor in the tumultuous waters of the healthcare system.

Nursing & caring for a patient with M.E. requires specific training as per criteria designed specifically for patients with ME. This is not a patient for the inexperienced Carer.

SOME QUESTIONS WORTH CONSIDERING FOR NURSES AND OTHERS OFFERING CARE

~

These are some of the things that you may need to consider:

- What do you know about Severe and Very Severe ME?
- Does the person need their own room, in a hospital setting?
- Does the person need special environmental provision in an outpatient setting?
- Does the person need care day and night and assistance with all areas of their life?
- Does anything they do have a potential after-affect that can affect them hours or days or weeks at a time?
- Can they move their limbs?
- Can they open their eyes or speak?

- Do they require assistance with a drink?
- Do they have any specific hypersensitivity to noise? How does that impact care?
- Do they have any special dietary, eating or feeding requirements?
- Do they need physical help in order to move?
- Do they need help getting into and pushing a wheelchair?
- Do they have a hoist?
- How do they transfer from their bed to their wheelchair and from their wheelchair to any other surface, for example the toilet, examination couch, another seat or is this not possible? What help is required?
- What help do they need getting to and using the toilet? Bathing? Showering?
- What aids do they need?
- Do they have a Catheter?
- Do they experience body pain?
- What degree of physical pain are they in?
- Do they experience Muscle fatigue? Muscle dysfunction?
- Do they have an inability to stand without support?
- Are they bed-bound for large portions of the day, or totally bed-bound?
- Do they have restricted mobility?
- Do they experience body spasms, paralysis, numbness, shaking?
- Do their muscles just stop working all of a sudden?
- Are their muscles able to hold them up?
- Do they blackout upon standing?
- Do they have poor spacial awareness?

- Do they bump into things?
- Can they bear physical contact? How do you approach this?
- Do they suffer from pins and needles, flowing and moving sensations?
- How does temperature affect them?
- Do they suffer from numbness that affects their ability to feel fully?
- Do they need someone around at all times because they are in danger of falling or hurting themselves?
- Are they completely immobile for large parts of the day, all the time, or does it vary?
- Are they in constant and severe pain?
- Do they need someone always available to help them within calling distance?
- Can they use/hold a buzzer?
- How do they summon you?
- Without ongoing assistance, day and night, would they get their basic needs met?
- Can they predict or determine how they will be in any one moment?
- Are actions reliable and repeatable?
- Does contact from other people have a post-exertional impact resulting in worsening symptoms?
- Does light hurt them?
- Do they have to have the curtains pulled, low lighting at best or complete darkness?
- Does heat or cold or both make them feel more ill?
- Do they run out of energy and feel even more ill with exacerbated symptoms after even small activity or movement?
- Have they developed a heightened awareness to

chemicals and odours leading them to feel nauseous, have a headache or other symptoms?
- Does their diaphragm ache and struggles with breathing?
- Do they get breathless quickly?
- Does the person use oxygen? How does this affect them?
- Do they have cognitive issues that affect memory, understanding and communication?

Make sure that you are aware of all that you need to know in order to provide correct care. Do not neglect a patient through ignorance of how their illness affects them and the help they need you to give.

96
SELF-REFLECTIVE QUESTIONS FOR PROFESSIONALS INVOLVED IN CARING

This book has tried to show how skilled and how challenging it is, yet how rewarding and important it is, to offer care and support to someone diagnosed with Severe ME and Very Severe ME.

To conclude this section on professional issues and advocacy, here are a few questions to stimulate reflection about your own knowledge, attitude, approach and practice.

1. WHAT ARE MY ATTITUDES AND BELIEFS ABOUT ME? HOW DO THEY AFFECT MY PRACTICE?

It is essential that you are aware of your attitudes, values and beliefs about this illness, as they will overtly or covertly impact your interactions.

2. DO I NEED TO ADAPT OR CHANGE MY APPROACH?

This will affect how you interact, what you see and what you discern as relevant and important.

- What is your normal approach to working with a client?
- Do you need to make any specific adjustments to maximise the success of any planned interaction, due to the nature and severity of illness?

3. Do I need to change my assumptions?

These may skew any decisions or judgements that you may have to make. What assumptions do you already have about ME?

4 Do I need to change my communication style?

This is key to any interaction. If you do not know how to be in the presence of someone with complex communication difficulties, you may make wrong assumptions, ignore their input, not understand how you are directly impacting them and not know how to approach them in the right way.

5. Do I need to change my expectations?

These need to be based on correct knowledge and awareness of the disease and how it affects the person. If you do not adjust your expectations to accommodate the way the symptoms impact and the experience of the person or if you expect more of the person than is possible, the interaction will be disastrous and the professional relationship put in jeopardy.

. . .

6. What do I specifically know about ME?

Write down the sum of your knowledge of ME:

- what you think it is
- how it affects people
- how it will impact your interaction and effectiveness in your role

7. What do I not know enough about in relation to Severe and Very Severe ME?

Be honest about any areas of knowledge that are cloudy or not known. Learn as much as you can from safe sources and from people themselves, through their descriptions, their films, their videos, their art and their written materials.

8. Do I specifically need to learn anything to improve my skills and knowledge?

Write a list of skills that you need to safely interact.

- Tick which ones you already have.
- How do you need to adapt them, if at all, when planning to interact with someone with Severe or Very Severe ME?
- What more do you think you need to be able to do?

9. What do I need to be more aware of, particularly in relation to my interactions and communication with

people with Severe ME or Very Severe ME?

Write a list of potential issues facing you concerning how you need to be, to prepare, to act, to speak, to move, to obtain information and approach contact.

10. What would a Risk Assessment entail in my role?

A Risk Assessment is critical to avoid harm and deterioration from any professional's engagement. We consider that a Risk Assessment should begin with understanding and knowledge of the person and the disease including any issues pertinent to that person's symptom experience. We believe that the risks of interacting need acknowledgment and due consideration, as well as any outcomes and recommendations made by professionals. There must be accountability and responsibility for engagement and recommendations made. The impact must be considered in advance and taken into account as much as possible.

11. Write 10 things that would improve your practice.

12. Do I need further training or experience in this area?

PART SEVEN: REMEMBERING THOSE WHO HAVE DIED

Welcome to the final part of this book! Here we take a moment to reflect upon all those we have known who have died. We have sadly known far too many wonderful people, who have died, sometimes very painfully. We cannot ignore or forget their suffering.

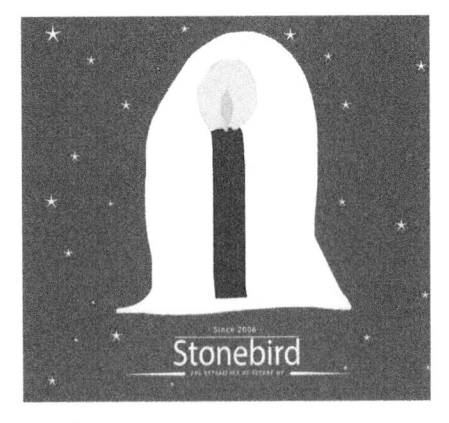

Yes! We will remember Yes! We will remember them Yes! We will always remember them

SEVERE MYALGIC ENCEPHALOMYELITIS, UNDERSTANDING AND REMEMBRANCE DAY, AUGUST 8TH: YES WE WILL REMEMBER

SEVERE ME UNDERSTANDING and Remembrance day, August 8th focuses on all the amazing people known and unknown, who have suffered horrendously, often for many, many years and who have died with ME.

Having known the wonderful young woman, now gone, whose idea it was to honour people with Severe ME by creating this special day on the anniversary of Sophia Mirza's birthday, we feel an extra special commitment to make this day a powerful recognition of all who have died.

We hold them in our hearts. We never forget them. The injustices and the sheer level of suffering they experienced can never be forgotten.

Their friendships and their memories deserve to be remembered. We also remember the people who loved and cared for them, the pain they witnessed, the losses, the struggles, the suffering they too experienced as they tried to get justice, give comfort and support, gain right medical input, speak out, to raise awareness of this devastating neurological disease, tragically neglected and ignored for decades.

Each person's loss, echoes through the whole ME community and brings an unhealable pain that they are no longer here and we affirm that all their loveliness, their passion for life, their commitment to truth, their individuality and their suffering will not have been in vain, will not be forgotten. They will be remembered.

So on August 8th every year, we take time to remember all the kindnesses, all the words of support, the gifts and encouragement that we have personally received, their amazing achievements, despite the tremendous, indescribable suffering. We hold them in our hearts particularly on the day and affirm that we will never forget them.

Their lives had meaning to so many, even if they were house and bed-bound, invisible to many in the outside world, they were not invisible to us.

∼

AND SO WE SAY, as we light a candle at 3pm on August 8th:

> Yes! We will remember
> Yes! We will remember them
> Yes! We will always remember them

99

DON'T LET US DOWN!

Our dear friend Kara Jane's song, 'Remember Us' from her new album 'It's Still ME', released on August 8th, Severe Myalgic Encephalomyelitis Understanding and Remembrance Day 2020, truly touches the soul.

This song is heartbreakingly beautiful. The words go right to the core of your being: *'You let me down, you let her down, you let him down, you let us down.'*

They play in your heart, still, long after the song has been played, hauntingly reminding you of the grief of so many lives lost, so many friends and others who have died tragically, painfully, with Severe ME, so many years wasted in endless agony and inability, so much suffering that it is unquantifiable, indescribable, ragged with pain.

So much denial, so much injustice, so much mistreatment, that it tears at our hearts. So many tortured moments remembered, as Kara sings, "you let me down".

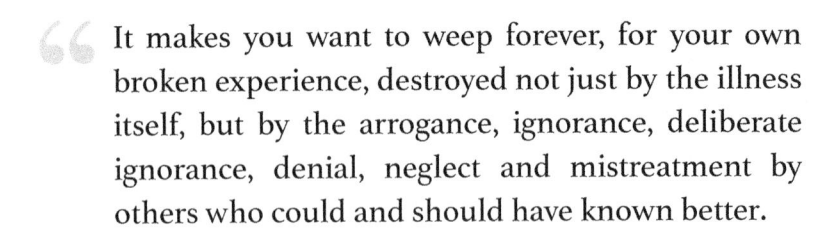

> It makes you want to weep forever, for your own broken experience, destroyed not just by the illness itself, but by the arrogance, ignorance, deliberate ignorance, denial, neglect and mistreatment by others who could and should have known better.

This song truly touches the soul. It reminds us of the beautiful lives lost, each precious, each harmed by the medical neglect of this serious neurological, multi-system impacting disease.

So many people have been let down.

As years go by the list of people who have died, gets added to.

Each year that Severe Myalgic Encephalomyelitis Understanding and Remembrance Day comes round, we cannot fail but to remember them. Nothing else will suffice.

We pray and hope that Kara is successful in raising the funds for a much needed Tissue Biobank to research and explore the medical reality of this disease and identify the underlying pathology. It may be the only way that we will finally get the consistent physiological answers that we need to be helped and recognised. Our voices indeed need to be heard and help, the right help, finally needs to be provided.

What a beautiful way to raise money for such an important provision.

We wish Kara every success in raising the money and really hope that others too will be deeply touched and moved particularly by this song that we now have written on our heart forever.

We ask then, who has let us down?

We ask then, how have they let us down? This is the answer.

. . .

WHO HAS LET US DOWN?

- Families who do not seek to truly understand and include.
- Friends who walk away, judge, blame or just get tired of you being too ill to connect with easily, as before.
- Neighbours who chose to ignore your needs because they are too inconvenient for them to be bothered with.
- Charities who support, in any way, the Biopsychosocial interpretation of ME in any form, by collaboration or validation or simply by not standing up against the misinformation and mistreatment of ME.
- Clinicians and other practitioners who chose to follow a psychosocial interpretation and agenda that completely denies the reality of the disease.
- GP's and other medical professionals who chose not to do home visiting to those unable to go to them.
- Anyone who says, this disease does not exist.
- Anyone who says, "but you look so well...."
- Anyone who ignores your reality.
- Anyone who choses to misuse the name Myalgic Encephalomyelitis and change its meaning from an Enteroviral Disease to a generalised fatigue state.
- Anyone who believes that there is no underlying pathology to the disease.
- Anyone who ignores paralysis is a very real symptom.
- Anyone who negates the reality of a person diagnosed with Severe ME and mistreats them as a consequence.

How have they let us down?

- Misinterpretation.
- Mistreatment.
- Misdiagnosis.
- Misunderstanding.
- Misinformation.
- Misdirection.
- Denial.
- Neglect.
- Collaboration with people who deny our reality and negate the disease.
- Lack of funding.
- Lack of reliable, repeatable, quality research.
- Denying the cause of the disease.
- Burying ME in a sea of poorly identified conditions.
- Not providing ongoing clinical support.
- Not teaching the correct information about the disease.
- Leaving patients neglected with little or no proof of the severity of their illness.
- Not adequately listening.
- Not believing.
- Not knowing up to date medical research and information.
- Poor research criteria.
- Ignoring patient input.
- Not creating a biomedical health pathway.
- Wrong reports.
- Self-justification.

- Self-importance.
- Ignorance.
- No treatment pathway.
- No cure.
- No hope.
- No justification for their behaviour towards us.
- Unkindness.
- Insensitivity.
- Carelessness.
- Disinterest.
- Too hard or difficult to be bothered with.
- Too much effort required.
- Laziness.
- Selfishness.
- Blame.
- Inadequacy.
- Incompetence.
- Failure to understand.
- Failure to reach out.
- Failure to connect.
- Failure to remain.
- Lack of commitment.
- Allowing people to be underfunded for basic living needs.
- Not creating special aids particularly pertinent to the experience.
- Ignoring key symptoms.
- Down playing the severity or experience.
- Excluding people.
- Ignoring the most ill leaving them to get on with it alone in isolation and separation, without the ability to speak up or help themselves.

- Leaving us without the pathology or knowledge we need to keep ourselves safe.
- Blame.
- Hostility.

It would be possible to go on and on with these lists but sadly they would get too long to remember the beginning of them.

We hope that you too are touched by Kara's song. 27 years of being let down, is for us, far too much. For others it is longer.

Still others take their lives because of the ignorance and the neglect and sheer intolerability of symptoms and circumstances.

Others die from the severity of their symptoms and the lack of knowledge of how to be with them and help them. This compounds the tragedy and pain of living with Severe and Very Severe ME or comorbid conditions.

The album has been available on all major platforms since August 8th 2020

WE REMEMBER: A REFLECTION FOR SEVERE ME DAY

∼

We remember them with kindness for it is important to honour the dead

We remember them with tenderness for we cared beyond imagining

We remember them with trepidation for we have to face our losses

We remember them with boldness for it takes courage remembering the pain

We remember them with sadness that they are no longer here with us

We remember them with frustration that they were not helped

We remember them with anger that they are gone

For we remember

All the hurt

All the denial

All the extremity of pain
All the neglect
All the harm
All the harrowing moments
All the suffering
All the grief
And we weep with gratitude
For their precious lives
For their tremendous personal strength
For their utmost conviction
For their forthrightness in speaking out
For their passion in life
For their compassion to others
In a hostile, empty world
We remember and give thanks
For who they were
And who they will always be
In our hearts

101

A TRAIL OF LOVE

∼

They leave a trail of love in your heart when they go,
Each one adding together to the many others
Who sing and dance and leave a path of memories
in your mind,
Till the whole is greater than the sum of the parts.
Wrapped in a special golden energy,
Their images dance within you.
Flashes of kindness, sadness, special words and deeds,
All meaningful, important somehow, precious,
Come back at unexpected moments,
Tip over into every day feelings,
Run riot with happiness and grief,
Blend your mood with loss and remembering,
Yet touch your life with an urgency
To live,
To feel,

To dance,
To express,
To be
Something,
Anything,
More than what you have been.
Whilst there is still time
Live,
Laugh,
Love,
Be
Present
Now
And recognise
The sacred space
That is your life
And always remember
How they have touched you,
How they have helped you,
How they have loved you too.

A THANK YOU TO A FRIEND WHO IS DYING

∼

I give thanks for all that you have been to me.
I give thanks for all that you have shared with me.
I give thanks for how knowing you has blessed my life.
I give thanks for all the hard-won moments of contact with you.
I give thanks for our special friendship, through all the difficult days.
I will never forget your kindness to me.
I will never forget your support and encouragement.
I will never forget your wise words to me.
I will never forget all the love we have shared between us.
I will never forget you, ever.........
You will always remain in my heart.

FOR MORE INFORMATION

∼

For much more information on how to care and find inspiration, please see Stonebird where there are a wide range of free care documents and information:

- **Caring For ME, a Pocketbook Course for Carers.**
  "We hope this will be a great life saver to many carers out there ...This book offers a caring and helping hand coming from a person of such experience and knowledge in the field. " 25% ME Group http://stonebird.co.uk/CARE/index.html
- **Notes for Carers An illustrated handbook packed full of practical tips, insights, guides and exercises.** http://stonebird.co.uk/Notes/index.html
- **Emily Collingridge's book**
- http://www.severeme.info
- **Voices from the shadows film**

- http://voicesfromtheshadowsfilm.co.uk
- **The ME show, Gary Burgess: podcast Episode 8**
- http://www.meassociation.org.uk/podcast/
- **25% ME Group**
- https://25megroup.org
- **The Grace Charity for ME**
- https://www.thegracecharityforme.org/prayer/
- For children: **The Tymes Trust**
- https://www.tymestrust.org
- **The North Carolina/Ohio ME & FM Support Group** https://www.facebook.com/groups/664421016959132/
- **Hope4ME & Fibro Charity**
- https://hope4mefibro.org/about/
- **ME Advocates Ireland**
- http://meadvocatesireland.blogspot.com/
- **Global Advocates 4 Myalgic Encephalomyelitis. GA4ME**
- https://artzstudios1.wixsite.com/globaladvocatesmeicc

AFTERWORD

∼

This is the fourth and last book. Completing it has been immensely challenging. I very much wanted to follow up my previous book, "*Notes For Carers*" with what I hope is a comprehensive Care Guide, especially for those who are new to caring. There is so much more though, still to say....!

Walking the dog this morning, I was reflecting upon how our situation is silent, fragile and complex beyond comprehension.

I was thinking about how my learning comes from that silence.

What is it all about? I was asking myself. This book, this life, this journey we are all on?

For me it is about continual learning, growing and developing my awareness, so that I can flow and be present rather than be distracted or unfocused and unaware.

The importance of the word "silence" just kept impressing itself on me.

For it is only in the silence that flows from your heart, I find, that you can listen with love, empathy and understanding.

It is only in the silence of your mind that you can be fully present to the other person without distraction or wishing you were some place else or busy doing something much more important or interesting.

And it is only in the silence of your being that you can be truly available to help.

Grace, presence and inner peace; ultimately, these proceed from the silence.

As does the greatest joy and connection.

May it be your guide, as it is mine.

ABOUT THE AUTHOR

My commitment to person-centred, values-based ways of being with people dates back to my work in the 1980's, alongside people who had a learning and a physical disability. I had no idea back then how the oppression and discrimination that I would encounter, much later, in the world of Severe/Very Severe ME, would be far worse than anything I had ever seen or could possibly have imagined.

It has led me, over decades, to fight for a proper medical service for people with ME. Learning how to be with someone in intense pain and suffering, for many years, in a posture of Partnership, has been the greatest privilege of my life.

I am an award winning Nurse with qualifications in Counselling, Coaching, Spiritual Care, Staff Training and Development, Experiential Learning and an MA in Moral, Personal and Spiritual Development.

This is my fourth book on Severe ME. For details of my other books please see Stonebird

https://stonebird.co.uk/

Printed in Great Britain
by Amazon